Tao Lin

TRIP

Tao Lin is the author of the novels *Taipei* and *Richard Yates* and *Eeeee Eee Eeee*, the novella *Shoplifting from American Apparel*, the story collection *Bed*, and the poetry collections *cognitive-behavioral therapy* and *you are a little bit happier than i am*. He was born in Virginia, has taught in Sarah Lawrence College's MFA program, and is the founder of Muumuu House.

TRIP

TRIP

PSYCHEDELICS,

ALIENATION,

AND CHANGE

Tao Lin

VINTAGE BOOKS
A Division of Penguin Random House LLC
New York

A VINTAGE ORIGINAL, MAY 2018

A portion of this work first appeared as "Beyond 'Existentialism'"
on *Vice* (www.vice.com) on July 8, 2014.

Page 309 constitutes an extension of the copyright page.

Library of Congress Cataloging-in-Publication Data
Names: Lin, Tao, 1983– author.
Title: Trip : psychedelics, alienation, and change / Tao Lin.
Description: New York : Vintage Books, 2018. | Includes bibliographical
references and index. | Identifiers: LCCN 2017041009 (print) |
LCCN 2017043462 (ebook)
Subjects: | MESH: McKenna, Terence K., 1946–2000. | Lin, Tao, 1983– |
Psychotropic Drugs—therapeutic use | Plant Extracts—therapeutic use | N,N-
Dimethyltryptamine—therapeutic use | Psilocybin—therapeutic use | Salvia |
Cannabis | United States | Personal Narratives
Classification: LCC RM315 (ebook) | LCC RM315 (print) |
NLM QV 77.2 | DDC 615.7/88—dc23
LC record available at https://lccn.loc.gov/2017041009

Vintage Books Trade Paperback ISBN: 978-1-101-97451-3
eBook ISBN: 978-1-101-97450-6

Book design by Anna B. Knighton

www.vintagebooks.com

Printed in India

10

CONTENTS

TRIP

INTRODUCTION

I learned of Terence McKenna (1946–2000) on September 14, 2012, the day after completing the main final draft of *Taipei*, my seventh book, third novel, and first book to include psychedelics. I was in my room, zombielike and depressed after embodying a "whatever it takes" attitude regarding amphetamines and other drugs and completing my novel. I had clicked a YouTube video in which Joe Rogan, whom I was vaguely aware of as the host of *Fear Factor*, was aggressively, excitedly talking about DMT, an illegal compound made by many species of plants and animals, including humans.

At one point Rogan began referencing someone in an "if you think *I* sound crazy, listen to this other guy" manner. He referred to Terence McKenna, a person who would smoke DMT and, within a minute, every time, find himself in an "unanticipated dimension" infested with "self-transforming machine elves" that spoke English and a kind of "visible language" while jumping in and out of his body, "running around chirping and singing." McKenna described these things, which he also called "fractal elves" and "jeweled self-dribbling basketballs," in a word as "zany." He speculated they were dead people in an "ecology of souls," humans from the future, or entities in a parallel world with their own hopes and problems.

The next week or so, alone in my room, which received no direct sunlight, I listened to McKenna make "small mouth noises," as he called human speech, on YouTube for probably thirty-plus hours—including in a ten-hour-and-twenty-three-minute, three-day workshop—with sustained, intrigued interest. I estimate this was twenty-five to twenty-seven more hours than I'd ever spent listening to an individual talk on YouTube. My unprecedented level of interest surprised me. McKenna seemed excited and delighted by topics I'd just finished expressing in my novel as sources of bleakness and despair and confusion—technology, drugs, human existence, the future.

He spoke on a myriad of what seemed gradually less like disparate interests than one purposed, interconnected, developing "web" of topics. He discussed consciousness, language, literature, art, memory, time, religion, dreams, octopi, math, aliens, biology, botany, shamanism, schizophrenia, psychotherapy, alienation, culture, sex, light, death, DNA, the *I Ching*, the internet, virtual reality, nanotechnology, artificial intelligence, family, fractals, feelings, science fiction, self-empowerment, and, at the center of it all, the impetus and sustaining force for the web's construction and elaboration, "the psychedelic experience," specifically the effects of psilocybin and DMT on humans.

His model of the universe had a singularity at the end—a mysterious attractor, pulling us to it—instead of at the beginning, as with the Big Bang, a theory he called "the limit test for credulity" because it asked one to accept the unlikeliest scenario possible, that everything appeared instantly from nothing for no reason. "If you can believe that, you can believe anything," said McKenna, taking something I'd encountered hundreds of times—and had always felt "nothing" toward—and successfully representing it to me, with the energizing suddenness of an epiphany, as a comical, egregious, eerie absurdity.

At a weekend workshop in December 1994, McKenna recalled some questions he'd had in 1961 as a fourteen-year-old: "What are we? Where did we come from? And where are we going?" His response—a reasonable one, he felt—was to check the cultural database. "Surely there are answers to these questions," he thought. He found that

> our best efforts are nothing more than half-completed stories told around the campfire. We don't actually know what our predicament is. We are up against a phenomenon which we can *barely* bring into focus in our cognitive sphere, and it's the phenomenon of our own existence. What does it mean? What does it mean, first of all, to be a biological creature—to be, as an animal—what is *that*?

And then what was that, embedded then in a culture with languages and aesthetic canons and cosmic theories? McKenna was unsatisfied with the conventional answers. But, beginning with *The Doors of Perception* (1954) by Aldous Huxley (1894–1963), he'd also been introduced, also at age fourteen, to "the whole array of consciousness-altering substances"—cannabis, LSD, DMT, psilocybin, mescaline—that in the past hundred years had "come into the toolbox of thinking Westerners." These substances, called psychedelics, put one in the metaphysical unknown by dissolving ideological, personal, and other boundaries. McKenna explained:

> All these things you might cling to—Catholicism, democratic ideals, Hasidism, Marxism, Freudianism—all of these

things are exposed as simply quaint cultural artifacts, painted masks and rattles assembled by people of good intent but clearly not great grasp of the situation. Well, I thought that that process of deconstruction of cultural reality would end in a kind of liberation of cynicism, where you become sort of *really* street smart, you know—nobody can put anything over on you, you've been there, you've done that. It turns out that that existential phase, which I reached at about age eighteen, is itself simply a place, along the way.

I think I reached that place when I was twenty or twenty-one, but in a vague, already-alienated way—I'd written an essay on existentialism when I was eighteen that concluded that people disagreed on what it was; I felt I didn't understand the Sartre I'd read; and I was unmoved by *The Stranger*, which I found melodramatic and unrelatable, though I also often found myself melodramatic and unrelatable—and I began to view it as "simply a place" maybe a year or two later. It was a place that didn't stimulate or comfort me anymore, but I remained there, even after, at twenty-seven, I had my first psychedelic experiences via psilocybin and LSD. I was still there after contemplating and describing those experiences for two years and feeling "done" with them, on some level, upon completing *Taipei*, which ended with a scene in which a character on psilocybin thinks he's dead.

Life still seemed bleak to me, as it had in evolving ways since I was thirteen or fourteen. I was chronically not fascinated by existence, which, though often amusing and poignant, did not feel wonderful or profound but tedious and uncomfortable and troubling. Life did seem mysterious, but increasingly only in a blunt, cheap, slightly deadpan, somehow unintriguing manner. As I aged, I seemed to become less curious why I was here, where I came from, and what would happen when I died. Psychedelics alone had not been enough to significantly affect my worldview. I required both psychedelics and McKenna—among other things, which I share in this book—to persuade and lure and charm and provoke me to depart the familiar and dead-end-like land of existentialism in an organized, sustained manner.

Before encountering McKenna, I'd felt only alienated, mostly, by the admittedly little I'd read, seen, and heard about psychedelics. People seemed to me superstitious, irrational, hyperbolic, dishonest, and/or incurious when discussing them, even and sometimes especially if they were advocating them. Not unexpectedly, people seemed satisfied to express and embody the same stereotypes—and embodying stereotypes is something I do too, an example being my "whatever it takes" mind-set—about psychedelics that had kept me away from them most of my life. Alienated from what others thought about them—and feeling like I'd confirmed to myself by writing *Taipei* that I had not been significantly affected by them—my interest in psychedelics dwindled and I became nearly as uninterested in them as I'd become uninterested in "the existential place."

After listening to McKenna talk for more than thirty hours, during which he spoke around as many words as are in a seven-hundred-page book, I became interested in psychedelics again and in new ways. I began to view them—and everything, including myself—within a context spanning from the unknown origins of the universe to when the sun formed in the Milky Way galaxy, through the emergence of biology and its development over three to four billion years on Earth from microorganisms to fish to amphibians to reptiles to mammals to primates to humans to *Homo sapiens*, around 300,000 years ago, until, finally, 15,000 to 25,000 years ago, the beginning of a brief transformation called history, which McKenna compared to the gestation period in the metamorphosis of a caterpillar to a butterfly, except instead of gaining wings as a specimen, we will be "turning ourselves inside out" as a species.

○

In June 2013, nine months after I encountered McKenna, *Taipei* was published. During my book tour I felt most engaged when people asked about psychedelics or McKenna, topics I'd mentioned in tweets. I told people I'd become more interested in psychedelic drugs than the drugs I'd focused on most in *Taipei* and other art—drawings, essays, movies—I'd released in the past three years. I was glad to distance myself from amphetamines, benzodiazepines, opiates, and MDMA because I felt they would, for me, lead to scarily more depression and anxiety. By explaining that my interests had changed, more people in the future would talk to me, I knew, about cannabis, psilocybin, LSD, DMT, salvia, and other psychedelics.

At Skylight Books in Los Angeles, I discussed McKenna's idea that "our map of the world is so wrong that where we have centered physics, we should actually place literature as the central metaphor that we want to work out from," as he explained in "Shamanology" (1984) in a quote I later taped to my wall and memorized and which continued: "Because I think literature occupies the same relationship to life that life occupies to death. . . . In the sense that a book is life with one dimension pulled out of it and life is something which lacks a dimension which death will give it. I imagine death to be a kind of release into the imagination in the sense that, for characters in a book, what we experience is an unimaginable dimension of freedom."

At Brazos Bookstore in Houston, a person asked during the Q&A after my reading if I'd smoked DMT. She was seated in the front row with a laser-like, unanxious gaze and looked like she was probably in high school. I said yes, but not enough else to cause anything except buzzing noises. She said she'd recently smoked DMT and asked if I'd read *The Cosmic Serpent* (1998). I said I'd just started it, actually, and asked how she'd found the somewhat obscure-seeming book, in which French anthropologist Jeremy Narby wrote about drinking ayahuasca with an Asháninca shaman while doing fieldwork in Peru for a doctoral degree. She said she'd found it randomly in a used bookstore. I was surprised she'd experimented with DMT and was talking to me about it in a bookstore in the presence of fifteen to twenty other people, including three of her friends—who seemed "dragged along," to some degree—and what seemed to be her mom.

In August, at a London bookstore and a Melbourne writers festival, I explained to audiences who'd ostensibly come to hear me discuss *Taipei* how, earlier in the month, I'd eaten psilocybin mushrooms, believed I was an alien occupying Tao Lin, sobbed for around an hour sitting on my bed, deleted parts of my internet presence, and thrown away my MacBook.

In September, back in my room, I considered how, in the year since discovering him, my interest in McKenna's ideas had not abated or weakened but invigoratingly endured and stabilized and expanded and deepened. This surprised me because part of me had expected to lose interest within weeks or months and revert, like many times before, somewhat sheepishly, to my vaguely existential worldview—in which I continually, if often halfheartedly, tried and failed to create and sustain my own meaning in life.

I was surprised again, another year later, in September 2014, when, after five months researching and writing a twelve-week, weekly column for *Vice* called Tao Of Terence—a goal of which, I stated in week 1, was to "spread Terence McKenna's memes"—I realized I was still interested in him and his ideas.

On some level, I had still suspected I'd become disillusioned, irrationally antagonistic, jaded, or indifferent—at least temporarily, for months or years—and as a side effect revert to feeling, again, "done" with psychedelics, but this hadn't happened.

A year and a half later, in February 2016, it still hasn't. It's been three and a half years since I discovered McKenna, and I'm ready to explain what I've learned and how I've changed. Besides to externalize, organize, contemplate, personalize, and share what has interested me most since completing *Taipei*, I have at least four other reasons for writing this book. The first two:

- To me, the world remains a terrible place, worthy of all the negative attributes I've called it in the past. But I'm now gratefully convinced it's also awe-inspiring and excitingly bizarre and complicatedly magical, a place of easily accessible wonder and pervasive, explorable, feelable mystery. I want to explain why.

- For reasons examined throughout this book, I've gradually realized that sustained, conscious effort is required—or at least strongly self-suggested—for me to not drift toward meaninglessness, depression, disempowering forms of resignation, and bleak ideologies like existentialism. This book is part of my effort.

☺

Trip is in eight chapters, with a long epilogue. In the first and second chapters, I examine McKenna's ideas and life. In the third chapter, I share my history with drugs, introduce my "recovery" and recovery, graph my drug history, and analyze my shift from pharmaceutical to psychedelic drugs.

In the fourth and fifth chapters, I examine my first three years and McKenna's three decades of experiences with psilocybin and DMT. I share accounts of my hedonistic, "alien sex," "leave society," exploratory, and paranoid psychedelic experiences. In the sixth chapter, I discuss *Salvia divinorum*, a plant introduced to modern people by the Mazatec of Central Mexico.

In the seventh chapter, I explore why psychedelics are illegal by investigating TV, magazine, newspaper, book, and government media; my experience serving on a "special narcotics" grand jury; McKenna's theory that they're illegal because they're "catalysts of intellectual dissent"; and our Goddess-worshipping, partnership past. In the eighth chapter, I fractally examine cannabis.

In the epilogue, I write about flying to California to meet Kathleen Harrison—whom McKenna married in 1976 and created children and a nonprofit organization with in 1978, 1980, and 1985—and be a student in her plant-drawing class.

WHY AM I INTERESTED IN HIM?

The first thing I noticed about him was his strange voice, which I felt aversion toward because my default state in 2012 while sober was an easily annoyed grumpiness. His nasally, slightly craggy, often high-pitched, sometimes low-pitched, slowish voice sounded surprisingly similar to the voice used by characters in *The Simpsons* who were "nerds"—low-charisma, socially clumsy, unathletic humans with thick glasses who spent most of their time with books and/or computers. I hadn't seen *The Simpsons*, which began seven years after McKenna started speaking publicly in recorded talks in 1982, in years and couldn't recall anyone else's voice reminding me of its "nerd voice." As I associated McKenna's unrushed cadence with his poignant ideas and reservedly cheerful, calmly skeptical, playfully self-aware, contemplative personality, my aversion dissipated and was quickly forgotten. Now I liked his style of talking for its distinctly noncommercial, I felt, oddness, its thorough enunciation and sometimes singsongy lilt. Now it seemed funny and auspicious to me that a person with this voice existed and was using it to share his extreme-seeming worldview to audiences of delighted, laughing, giggling people. I enjoyed McKenna's triangulating deviations into stand-up comedy and, as I experienced it, "fiction"—sentences I'd feel similarly stimulated and moved by if I read them in a short story or novel, like when he said, in a 1998 talk:

> The toughest thing to figure out is relationships. It is the yoga of the West. But it's harder than yoga. I'm fifty-two, merely—and I don't feel greatly wiser in this area than I felt at twenty-four. And, you know, I've had a marriage, I've had a divorce, I've been single, I've had long-term relationships, short-term relationships, on and on and on.

He seemed always partially talking to himself but was also teacher-like, often unpromptedly defining and verbally footnoting terms, names, and historical events. "I represent to myself—and I hope to convince you of this—radical ideas, innovative ideas, even peculiar ideas, but not loose or preposterous ideas," he said in one talk. His language was a mix of idiomatic, literary, poetic, popular, obscure, crass, ventriloquial, scientific, and academic. "Notice that I use big words," he said when asked in 1992 why, as an assiduous, long-term promoter of illegal drugs, he wasn't in jail. "I don't try to boil it down to a shoutable slogan, like 'Turn on, tune in, drop out'? Uh-uh, that—then they come, they come. So that's one possibility—that, simply, if you are defined in their eyes as an intellectual, then they automatically put you in the harmless category and send resources elsewhere." Except for a title and sometimes a list of topics, his talks, which were forty to ninety minutes and usually ended with thirty to sixty minutes of Q&A, and workshops (connected talks over multiple days) were improvised. They employed a wandering, exploratory form, like the tunnel an ant might create by entering a cube of sand at one point and exiting at another, with the cube representing McKenna's knowledge on a chosen subject and the tunnel, exiting in a manner seeming inevitably abrupt, being the content of the talk. McKenna's disembodied voice creakily emanated from the 1980s and 1990s, through the internet, into my room—which often felt cave-like in late 2012—and I learned scattered details about his life and ideas:

- He insisted the world was made of language. Not the thoughts of God, quarks, electromagnetic wave packets, planets, or stars but language. He called this "the primary fact that has been overlooked."

- He'd been attracted, since he was a small child, to the weird, which led him to psychedelics—the ultimate, he felt, in weird. "Weird is the compass heading," he said.

- He called himself "a hardheaded rationalist" and seemed more earnest and sophisticated and undeluded than anyone I'd absorbed this much information from on nonmaterial topics like consciousness and imagination. He had arrived at his conclusions—that there was "confounding, paranormal material" in the psychedelic experience, that humans were near the end of time—through skepticism and disbelief.

- He distinguished himself from the New Age, which he called "a flight from the psychedelic experience," and various other contemporary groups attracted to occult and mystical topics. "I say this as a reasonable person," he said in 1992. "I want to keep stressing that. I won't sit at the same table as the channelers, and the people who have good news about Atlantis, and all of this stuff."

- Despite being extra-rational, he was also optimistic. This surprised me because I associated rational thinking with pessimism, or at least a wan, slightly feigned sort of optimism. McKenna was energetically optimistic. He called himself "a resolute optimist of a complicated sort." In one talk, he asked if there was "any reason why people of analytical intelligence, who are connected up to the facts of the matter about the state of the world, should hope." He observed that the conventional wisdom was "basically no," then explained why, in his view, "yes."

- He went to the gym as "psychedelic training"—to improve his ability to explore the unknown and bring back useful information.

- He'd "scoured India and other places" and been underwhelmed in terms of spiritual teachers—no one had shown him anything close to what psychedelics delivered reliably—and he was "not willing to climb aboard the Buddhist ethic because Buddhism says suffering is inevitable," which was "not a psychedelic point of view." Religions that had "made meditation the centerpiece of their ontology," like Mahayana Buddhism, were, he felt, nihilistic. This surprised me, because, at first mindlessly associating McKenna with the term "hippie," I had expected him to automatically regard Eastern philosophies—in a manner belying, I had always vaguely felt, some amount of mindlessness—as wise and praiseworthy.

- He argued, in a manner I found compelling and revelatory, that nature was not, as Sartre said, "mute," but that, obviously, it was people who were deaf. "The myth of our society is the existential myth that we are cast into matter, that we are lost in a universe that has no meaning for us, that we must make our meaning," he said in a 1998 workshop on alchemy. "This is what Sartre, Kierkegaard, all those people are saying, that we must make our meaning. It reaches its most absurd expression in Sartre's statement that nature is mute."

- He seemed to exclude nothing from his model building—the early internet and prehistoric shamanism, quantum physics and romantic love, Saharan rock art and the Hubble Space Telescope, Taoism and Riane Eisler.

As I solitarily and passively and sometimes distractedly—and also sometimes, at this point, a little skeptically but decreasingly so as I gradually realized the depth and carefulness of his words—assimilated all this and other atypical information from McKenna, I became, in the weeks and months after discovering him, especially interested in his ideas on ideas.

HE DIDN'T BELIEVE ANYTHING

McKenna stressed he deliberately didn't believe anything—even his own theories. "My technique, which I recommend to you, is don't believe anything," he said. "If you believe in something, you are automatically precluded from believing its opposite." Belief was a "self-limiting function," a "stultifying force." McKenna's disbelief was not due to apathy, cynicism, or stubbornness but determination, as he explained in "Gathering Momentum for a Leap" (1994):

> I have been vehemently accused by people who didn't understand me of not believing in anything. I *don't* believe in anything. This is not a statement of existential hopelessness for which you should light a candle for me at night. It's a strategy for not getting bogged down in some weird trip. After all, what is the basis for believing anything? I mean, you have to understand: You're a monkey. In some kind of a biological situation where everything has been evolved to serve the economy of survival—this is not a philosophy course. So belief is a curious reaction to the present at hand. It isn't to be believed; it's to be *dealt* with—experienced and modeled.

He was clear and persistent on this—"I would entertain any idea, but believe in nothing"; "I don't believe in belief"; "My anti-ideological stance makes it very important to believe nothing," he said in 1989, 1994, and 1996—and to me it was a central, vital, exciting aspect of his thinking, but many people, I found, seemed to ignore, overlook, or, for whatever reason, choose not to engage with or acknowledge it. "He believed wholeheartedly in the stories he told," wrote Andy Letcher egregiously in *Shroom* (2007) near the end of an error-ridden, partially dismissive chapter on McKenna, two pages after I wrote "this guy doesn't get McKenna" in the margins, for example.

HE WAS AGAINST GURUS

McKenna traveled the planet telling groups of people his ideas, including on what to ingest and how to save the world—an arguably guru-like activity—but, in most other ways, he was distinctly and severely not like a guru. "Avoid gurus, follow plants," he advised. "I think: no method, no guru, no teacher. Nobody has a handle on this; nobody understands. All these esoteric schools are the dealings of beady-eyed priests." He was "against any group who keeps secrets." He called secret-keeping "a bad habit" and "a way of controlling people." He promoted guru-defeating, self-empowering ideas that the mushroom told him, like: "For one human being to seek enlightenment from another is like a grain of sand on the beach seeking enlightenment from another."

Another way he was unguru-like can be found in a forty-minute five-second video on YouTube titled "A Conversation with Terence McKenna and Ram Dass (1992)" in which Dass, seated at a table with McKenna, said, "My mantra is the Gandhi line 'My life is my message.'" After nine seconds, during which they self-consciously, I felt, busied their mouths (McKenna with fork, Dass with cup), McKenna said:

> I think I'm at a lower level. Because I'm very aware that, um—I have to struggle to say "My life is my message." I would almost rather say "My message is my message. Please don't look at my life because I'm a fallible human being and I'm constantly fucking up."

"But, you see how that weakens your message?" said Dass.

McKenna answered with an anecdote: He once told Leo Zeff, the psychologist who pioneered the use of LSD and MDMA in psychotherapy, that Zeff was finished, was "baked." McKenna, however, was not; he was "half-baked," he told Dass, then laughed mildly. "And I hope that the rest of my life will finish the baking process," he said, turning to his food.

For me, this strengthened his message, gave his ideas an evolving, collaborative, discussable quality.

HE POINTED ME BACK TO MYSELF

McKenna promoted one thing arguably more than psychedelics: the felt presence of immediate experience. "No one knows how it is that I can command my hand to make a fist and that it will do that," he said in "Eros and the Eschaton" (1994). "I mean, that's mind over matter. That's the violation of every scientific principle in the books. And yet it is the most trivial experience any of us have; we expect to command our body." He called the body "the nexus of the mystery of life." While explaining his worldview, he sometimes paused to recommend that I focus on my own experiences, that I empower myself by creating culture based on my highs and plans and fears, my friends and body and history.

He was adamant and funny on this. Despite earning his income by sharing and explaining his ideas, he stressed that people should not listen to him. In one talk, he said "the mystery" was "best served by silence and contemplation"; then, changing tone, he said, "The problem is, you know, it's just hell on your bank account if you're a professional lecturer. So we drop down a level, to raving and ranting." Changing tone again, he elaborated in earnest: "But all of these things are provisional and literalistic. Nowhere is it writ large that the minds of higher primates are going to hold a simulacrum of reality."

In "Appreciating Imagination" (1994), responding to an audience member whose question was inaudible in the recording I heard, McKenna said, "Well, I hate to tell you this, but I would *NEVER* do what you are doing." This was the only instance in his verbal oeuvre where I felt the need to both italicize and use all-capital letters, and I felt it confidently, though it was not spoken loudly. This followed:

MCKENNA: This may be the ultimate teaching.

AUDIENCE: [laughter]

MCKENNA: Do not *ever again* spend money to see me. [In a slightly asided voice, laughing a little] Uh, my god, how much income is going down the drain as the ultimate oral empowerment is given?

AUDIENCE MEMBER: This is entertainment!

MCKENNA: [loud laughter] Well, okay, as long as you take it as entertainment, that's fine.

I took his talks as nourishment that was synergistically entertaining, that made me mentally and physically smirk, smile, grin, snicker, chuckle, chortle, and laugh while informing me in a non-boring, challenging manner on seemingly everything. Like a friendly, quick-witted, college-less meta-professor, he took the most interesting pieces, the glinting memes, from each subject— geology, physics, molecular biology, harmony and counterpoint— and shared them with me in a concise and original manner.

HE VIEWED IDEAS AS MEMES

McKenna defined a meme as "the smallest unit of an idea that still has coherency" and said he was very conscious of creating and spreading them during his talks. Madonna, socialism, yellow sweaters, rainbow-colored dreadlocks, DMT elves, and "the felt presence of immediate experience" were all memes, which were to ideology as genes were to biology. McKenna compared the ideological environment to a rain forest. "Launch your meme boldly and see if it will replicate—just like genes replicate, and infect, and move into the organism of society," he said in "Shamanism, Alchemy, and the 20th Century" (1996). "And, believing as I do that society operates on a kind of biological economy, then I believe these memes are the key to societal evolution."

Previously, in the cultures and subcultures I was part of or aware of existing around me—on the internet, in the media, and in the literary world—the word "meme" seemed to refer almost exclusively to photos and GIFs, sometimes with a small amount of overlaid text, that circulated online for the purpose of humor. I gladly supplemented that definition of "meme" with McKenna's broader, older usage of the word, which biologist Richard Dawkins invented in the 1970s.

As I continued listening to McKenna—who in one talk called himself "a meme replicator"—with varying amounts of attention, I noticed he had different definitions than most people for other words also. These words seemed mostly to be common abstractions that I'd always suspected people to be using with unexamined or deliberate vagueness, for rhetorical and commercial purposes. For some of these words, I felt I was finally encountering meanings I could understand and add to my mental dictionary.

TRUTH

Before McKenna, "truth" was a word I avoided earnestly using and tended to distrust and gloss over when others used it. Like the word "real," which McKenna also helped me to finally confidently define—" 'Real' is a distinction of a naïve mind, I think; we're getting beyond that," he said in "Techno-Pagans at the End of History" (1998)—people seemed to use the word "true" to externalize their mental hierarchies in which certain feelings, preferences, behaviors, beliefs, and lifestyles were ranked above others. Now truth seemed obviously to be a provisional, relative concern. Something could be "true enough." McKenna explained: "I'm sure some of you have heard me recall the situation where Wittgenstein was raving about something and one of his students said, 'But is it the truth?' And he said, 'Well, it's true enough.'"

HISTORY

Besides redefining the word "history" for me, McKenna also successfully interested me in learning about human history. Instead of a subject in school involving wars and treaties and generals, or the study of the past of any topic, history was now also a birth-like, 15,000-year transformation occurring late in biology on certain planets to certain species—a "nearly instantaneous transition" beginning with "animals kept in balance by natural selection" and ending with "the transcendental object at the end of time." History, in McKenna's view, was not "a trendlessly fluctuating process," nor a phase, to be continued for millions of years, but a phase *shift*, of which humans were only decades or centuries from the end—a possibility I'd never suspected and from which I now derived awe, mental stimulation, and meaning.

IMAGINATION

No longer a vaguely childish-seeming, fantasy-related abstraction that I associated mostly with poets and Disney, imagination became *the* imagination—a dimension outside time that was "accessible only to the degree that one can decondition oneself from the history-bound cognitive systems that have carried one to this point," explained McKenna. Realer and larger than the universe, the imagination was where bone flutes, ivory figurines, novels, sonatas, airports, dance moves, nuclear weapons, and computer games—captured by human consciousness and downloaded into matter—came from and where we, as individuals and a species, were going.

ALIENATION

I used to associate alienation mostly with sadness and meekness. I viewed it as a personal issue I could possibly overcome with regular exercise and more social contact. I'd encountered its political meaning in middle school through "punk music," as I examine in the third chapter, but in college it became more of a melancholic thing. After McKenna, my alienation regained the earlier meaning, became shared and justified. Instead of a glum, demoralizing, indirectly satisfying sensation, alienation now seemed once again action-oriented and hope-filled and analysis-demanding. It indicated something about my relationship with society. In "The World and Its Double" (1993), when his children were fifteen and twelve, McKenna said:

> The reason we feel alienated is because the society is infantile, trivial, and stupid. So the cost of sanity in this society is a certain level of alienation. I grapple with this because I'm a parent. And I think anybody who has children, you come to this realization, you know—what'll it be? Alienated, cynical intellectual? Or slack-jawed, half-wit consumer of the horseshit being handed down from on high? There is not

much choice in there, you see. And we all want our children to be well-adjusted; unfortunately, there's nothing to be well-adjusted *to*.

COMPLEXITY

"Complexity" used to be a somewhat mundane word, an antonym for simplicity. I was perpetually unsure if I wanted more or less in my life. Sometimes I admired and strove for complexity, but, on average, and increasingly, I seemed to prefer simplicity, maybe because it felt less stressful and crazed. Now complexity, which McKenna also called novelty, was the featured element of two crucial-seeming laws of nature that I'd never consciously acknowledged or heard of before. The first was "so obvious" it had "never been embraced as a general and dependable principle," said McKenna in 1994: As the universe ages, it complexifies. The second was that this process, in which previously achieved complexity is used to create more complexity, accelerates.

PSYCHEDELIC

Before McKenna, I associated the word "psychedelic" (which I didn't know meant "mind-manifesting") with a kind of vaguely hedonistic mindlessness. I more than half-believed the stereotypes I'd absorbed throughout my life about psychedelic drugs—that they caused insanity and out-of-control behavior and were hazardous and uninteresting. People on psychedelics, when not going insane, seemed to laze or frolic or dance in fields and not worry or think about anything but only (somewhat pointlessly, I'd always felt) look at things, which they usually described as geometric. Now I associated psychedelics with language, time, emotion, change, mystery, sanity, nature, compassion, learning, awe, problem-solving, the unconscious, and the unknown. "Living psychedelically is trying to live in an atmosphere of continuous unfolding of understanding," said McKenna in "Psychedelic Society" (1984). "So that every day you know more, and see into things with greater depth, than you did before."

In this chapter I've described McKenna's voice, shared what I learned early on about him, considered his meta-ideas, and examined his unusual definitions for six words. One reason I chose this mediumly discursive approach—to answering why I'm interested in McKenna—is to simulate my encounter with him in the last four months of 2012. Another reason is because it has increasingly been my view of his oeuvre that "no part is first and no part last," "every part supports the whole just as much as it is supported by the whole," and "even the smallest part cannot be fully understood until the whole has been first understood," as Arthur Schopenhauer (1788–1860), who, like McKenna, stressed experience via the body as the sole source of knowledge, wrote in 1818 in the preface to his main work. With this in mind, a sampler-like, many-parted, meme-studded method of teaching McKenna's worldview seemed most desirable.

But now I want to provide an opposite, balancing experience with a chronological narrative of McKenna's life, which is another reason why, besides his ideas, I'm interested in him.

TERENCE MCKENNA'S LIFE

The public story of Terence McKenna's life—as told in thousands of sentences and anecdotes from his talks and interviews, his essays "I Understand Philip K. Dick" (1991) and "Among *Ayahuasqueros*" (1992), his memoir *True Hallucinations* (1993), scattered mentions of him by his children and Kathleen Harrison, tens of newspaper and magazine articles on him, and around 20 percent of his brother Dennis's memoir *The Brotherhood of the Screaming Abyss: My Life with Terence McKenna* (2012)—would be, if collected into one place, around a five-hundred-page book, which, if it existed, could be titled *One Version of Terence McKenna's Life*. The following is my sixteen-page, ten-part biography of McKenna. It begins with an epigraph.

The world which we perceive is a tiny fraction of the world which we *can* perceive, which is a tiny fraction of the perceivable world.

—TERENCE MCKENNA, 1987, Los Angeles

1. PAONIA

Terence Kemp McKenna was born on November 16, 1946, in a one-hotel town in Colorado named Paonia. "They wanted to name it Peony but didn't know how to spell it," he said in an interview with *Omni* magazine in 1993. "In your last year of high school, you got your girlfriend pregnant, married her, and went to work in the coal mines. An intellectual was someone who read *TIME*."

It's unknown if Terence read *Time*, but he did, at least once, read *Life*. The May 13, 1957, issue included a first-person narrative, "Seeking the Magic Mushroom," in which R. Gordon Wasson (1898–1986) wrote about becoming, with photographer Allan Richardson, in a ceremony in Oaxaca with María Sabina (1894–1985), a Mazatec *curandera*, "the first white men in recorded history to eat the divine mushrooms." They "saw visions" and "emerged from the experience awestruck." The article included watercolor paintings of the seven known types of psilocybin-containing mushroom; the last painting, of five palely golden mushrooms, had this caption: "First discovered in Cuba in June 1904, *Stropharia cubensis* Earle grows on cow dung in pastures."

In this way, appearing bluntly in a mainstream magazine via the clear, lyrical, restrained prose of a New York banker, the mushroom introduced itself with characteristic charm and brashness to the McKenna brothers. In his 2012 memoir, Dennis, who was six, remembered Terence, who was ten, waving the magazine at their mom, following her as she did housework, demanding to know more. "But of course she had nothing to add," wrote Dennis.

Growing up, Terence wore thick bifocal glasses. He subscribed to the *Village Voice* and *Evergreen Review*—a literary magazine that published Kerouac, Burroughs, and others from 1957 to 1973—and collected fossils. "We would find dinosaur bones and two-hundred-million-year-old clam shells and stuff," he said in a talk in Manhattan in 1998. "And when I finally figured out that a million years is *a thousand years a thousand times*, it was like an epiphany." At age eleven or twelve, he began collecting insects and building model rockets, an interest his dad, who owned a plane and enjoyed flying, encouraged. He ordered butterflies and beetles from listings in the back of *Science News*. On weekends, his dad helped him build and launch solid-fuel rockets.

Over time, his weirder interests—drugs, magic, "the more obscure backwaters of natural history and theology"—came to dominate his attention. "There's something going on here for sure," he said to himself after reading *The Doors of Perception*, Aldous Huxley's seventy-one page account of his first mescaline trip. To the despair of their parents, Dennis shared Terence's interests, which, beginning in the early 1960s, because their dad sometimes brought home "sci-fi pulp mags," also included science fiction—most influentially *Star Maker* (1937) by Olaf Stapledon and *Childhood's End* (1953) and *The City and the Stars* (1956) by Arthur C. Clarke—which Terence later called his "entry drug." They wanted "answers to the ultimate questions," wrote Dennis in *The Brotherhood of the Screaming Abyss*, and were dissatisfied by the "shallow answers" provided by their Catholic faith.

To their parents, their most troubling interest was psychedelic drugs. Their mom, who'd introduced Terence to Huxley with *The Art of Seeing* (1942), was more receptive than their dad, with whom it was impossible to rationally discuss "drugs." A World War II veteran, he viewed alcohol as benign but felt cannabis, LSD, and heroin were all "intrinsically bad," wrote Dennis, who observed that their dad, with whom Terence had "ongoing contentious conversations" and "screaming matches" about drugs and other topics, "made the mistake of seeing evil as a moral quality imbued in the substances, not a product of how they were used."

2. CALIFORNIA

In 1963, when he was sixteen and the population of Paonia, at around 1,100, was near its lowest since the 1930s, Terence convinced his parents to let him move to California. He lived with an uncle and aunt in Los Altos, then a family friend in Lancaster, where he finished high school.

In 1965, he was admitted to UC Berkeley's Tussman Experimental College, a new program—replacing the first two years of curriculum for 150 of Berkeley's entering undergraduates—in which students created their own reading lists and weren't graded. He studied ecology, resource conservation, and shamanism, which was, he said in 1994, "about the felt presence of immediate experience in the absence of theory." Near the end of 1966, his mom and Dennis visited him, and he convinced his mom to smoke hash. She felt "so wracked with guilt, and so afraid of how furious Dad would be if he ever found out she'd actually gotten stoned with her sons, she couldn't really let herself go and enjoy the experience," wrote Dennis.

In early 1967, Terence smoked DMT. Compared to cannabis and LSD, both of which he'd encountered in 1965 and had been powerful in transforming his personality, DMT was of a different order of experience, raising questions that he felt science and philosophy needed to examine. By the end of his second year of college, his library had more than a thousand books. He lived in a three-story communal building on Telegraph Avenue in a room that became "a sort of informal salon where people would show up to get loaded and stay to hear him rant," wrote Dennis, who visited him in July of that year. "He often had a receptive audience of very stoned listeners hardly able to speak or move while he regaled them."

Terence worked that summer, the Summer of Love, mounting butterflies at the California Academy of Sciences. That fall, he paused his studies to travel with a girlfriend to India, Nepal, and elsewhere. His relationship ended during the trip and then, in Jerusalem, he met Kathleen Harrison, who was born on Catalina Island off the coast of Los Angeles and was also traveling and had smoked DMT even earlier than Terence—in 1966 as a freshman at UC Santa Cruz, when a friend offered her a DMT-laced joint, which they shared before entering a harpsichord concert. In 2013, Harrison described this brief encounter: "I wrote my mom a postcard from Jerusalem in 1967 that said 'I just met the weirdest person I've ever met, but I suspect he's going to have some kind of influence on my life.' "

Continuing his travels, Terence went south to Mombasa and rode a freighter to the Seychelles, an archipelago nine hundred miles from the east coast of Africa, to focus on writing. He planted cannabis seeds when he arrived, telling himself he would smoke the grown plants when he finished writing his book. "According to a story Terence would later tell, when that day came he got totally baked and realized what he'd written was terrible," wrote Dennis. Staying on Silhouette Island an extra month, smoking cannabis daily, he rewrote the book.

3. NEW YORK CITY

Months later, in fall 1968, Terence was in New York City failing to interest publishers in his book, which he would describe twenty-five years later as "a rambling, sophomoric, McLuhan-esque diatribe that was to die a bornin', fortunately" and was titled *Crypto-Rap: Meta-Electrical Speculations on Culture*. Seated, as he described in a scene in *True Hallucinations*, at an outdoor restaurant in Central Park with his friend Vanessa, whom he'd met in Berkeley, Terence discussed a startling idea his brother—"some sort of genius"—had that "some hallucinogens work by fitting into the DNA."

Vanessa, the only person he knew in the city, was from the Upper East Side. Terence said the political revolution had become "too murky a thing to put one's hope in." He called DMT "the most interesting unlikelihood" in their lives and wondered if they should "stop fucking around and go off and grapple with the DMT mystery." Which meant going to the Amazon. But Vanessa already had plans in Australia. "And I am committed to this hash thing in Asia in a few months," said Terence, "for who knows how long?"

4. ASIA

Terence lived in Nepal, smuggling hashish and, because of his interest in Tibet's indigenous, pre-Buddhist, shamanistic religion, studying the Tibetan language until late August 1969, when U.S. Customs intercepted one of his Bombay-to-Aspen shipments. Traveling under "the dramatic assumption," he wrote in *True Hallucinations*, that "international police agencies" were looking for him, he wandered through Southeast Asia viewing ruins and eastwardly crossed the Indonesian archipelago collecting butterflies.

In early 1970, he returned to city life, living in Hong Kong,

Taipei, and Tokyo, where he taught English. In the Berkeley hills, meanwhile, that summer, wildfires destroyed his friend's house that was storing his library and art collection. Terence obtained a false Australian passport and flew to Vancouver, Canada, where he lived for three months, during which (1) he and Dennis and two friends planned a trip to La Chorrera, a town in Colombia, in search of *oo-koo-hé*—a DMT-containing plant preparation they'd learned of from the June 25, 1969, issue of *Botanical Museum Leaflets*—and (2) his mom, who'd survived breast cancer five years earlier, died at age fifty-seven of bone cancer.

5. LA CHORRERA

In southern Colombia in early February 1971, Terence, Dennis, and now three friends (Vanessa, Ev, and Dave) encountered a large specimen of *Stropharia cubensis* sprouting from old cow manure in a meadow. At the suggestion of his companions, Terence ate the mushroom. "The eerie sense that some other dimension or scale of being had intersected with the bright tropical day lasted only a few minutes," he wrote in *True Hallucinations*. It was "unlike any feeling" he could recall. On February 21, after living with a Witoto tribe for almost a week, during which they hired two boys to help them carry their things, including a kilo of unexpectedly gained cannabis and a fiberglass butterfly net, then walking through the jungle for four days, they arrived at La Chorrera, where they found *Stropharia cubensis* growing on a large pasture where white cattle grazed.

On the night of March 4, two weeks later, deviating from the plan to spend three months "slowly getting to know the botanical and social environment of the Witoto" in service of finding *oo-koo-hé*, which seemed heavily taboo, the McKenna brothers performed "the experiment at La Chorrera." Using harmine from *Banisteriopsis caapi*, psilocybin from *Stropharia cubensis*, the body, a kind of singing, and the principles of superconductivity and harmonic resonance, they tried to intercalate psychoactive compounds into the rungs of neural DNA in order to create the philosopher's stone, or, as Terence in *True Hallucinations* quoted Dennis's journal entry from that day, "four dimensions captured and delineated in three."

The experiment was successful and not. It did not create a hyperdimensional object—the soul was not concretized—but it did, over weeks, seem to cause these unusual phenomena: sibling telepathy, cognitive hallucination, a teaching voice in the brothers' heads, mental phone calls decades through time, a UFO sighting containing its own debunking. Terence didn't sleep for nine days, during which he watched over Dennis, who "alternated between calmness and long harangues on a supra-cosmic scale," claiming he'd been smeared across the universe and was incrementally returning—condensing to the galaxy, the solar system, Earth, his extended family, and his sibling dyad before realizing he was Dennis. Ev, Terence's girlfriend, remained sympathetic, but the brothers' other friends did not. "Everyone thought that everyone else was crazy," wrote Terence in *True Hallucinations*.

On March 21, in his first journal entry in weeks, Terence wrote that the past few weeks had been "seemingly made of so many times, places, and minds" that "a rational chronicle" had been "impossible." Dennis flew home to Colorado on March 29, and on April 13, Terence returned to Berkeley. In July, he and Ev returned to La Chorrera, where the mushroom was less abundant than in February. They gathered spore prints and brought them to the States.

6. MUSHROOMS AND MARRIAGE

Five years later, in January 1976, *Psilocybin: Magic Mushroom Grower's Guide* by O. T. Oss and O. N. Oeric with drawings by Kat was published by And/Or Press. The sixty-four-page book began with a Wasson quote on finally knowing "what the ineffable is" and "what ecstasy means." Written by the McKenna brothers under pen names, it told how to grow and preserve *Stropharia cubensis*—"the starborn magic mushroom"—and featured eleven drawings of the mushroom in different contexts, including a life-cycle diagram, glass-jarred, and cosmic.

It was the brothers' second co-written book. The first, *The Invisible Landscape: Mind, Hallucinogens, and the I Ching*, had been published the previous year; in 229 pages, including an appendix of mathematical equations, it had examined what happened at La Chorrera within a shamanic framework, introduced a holographic theory of mind, and presented Timewave Zero, a model of history viewing time as a fractal phenomenon with an end. *The Invisible Landscape* had quickly gone out of print.

Psilocybin went through printings quickly. In the preface to its expanded 1986 edition, Terence wrote that more than a hundred thousand copies had been sold and that probably more people were "involved in a religious quest using psilocybin than ever before in history." A year before the guide was first published, in spring 1975, after he and Ev had separated, Terence and Kathleen Harrison met again. Eight years had passed since their Jerusalem meeting.

They became lovers that summer, moved to Hawaii that fall, and the next spring, in 1976, three months after the guide was published, traveled to Peru, where, over seven weeks, they experienced five days of cramped boat travel; equipped themselves against insects in Iquitos; found eighty-eight-year-old Manuel Córdova-Rios (the subject of the 1971 book *Wizard of the Upper Amazon*), who recommended Juana Gonzales Orbi; flew 334 miles to Pucallpa; failed to locate Orbi; met Don Fidel Mosombite; and, in the last three weeks, drank ayahuasca five times. They brought two kilograms of concentrated ayahuasca, which took three days to make, back to the suburban community in Berkeley where they now lived. Seven months later, on November 22, 1976, six days after Terence turned thirty and when Kathleen was twenty-eight, they married.

7. CONSULTING

In the early 1980s, living in Occidental, California, a town in Sonoma County as small as Paonia, with Kathleen and their children, Finn and Klea, born in April 1978 and December 1980, Terence began giving talks at Esalen Institute and elsewhere. "Usually the shaman is an intellectual and is alienated from society," he said at the Lilly/Goswami Conference on Consciousness and Quantum Physics in 1982. "You have to take seriously the notion that understanding the universe is your responsibility, because the only understanding of the universe that will be useful to you is your own understanding," he said at Shared Visions in Berkeley in 1983. He appeared repeatedly on a late-night Los Angeles radio show called "Something's Happening" to discuss psychedelics. How did this start? A 1993 interview with *tripzine* offered one answer:

> **INTERVIEWER**: So you lived on the royalties of the *Magic Mushroom Grower's Guide* alone?

TERENCE: And something which we should probably describe as "consulting."

INTERVIEWER: I see. [laughs]

TERENCE: [laughs loudly]

INTERVIEWER: [regaining composure] Well, I guess that's what I was shooting for with that question.

TERENCE: Yes, there was a lot of "consulting" in the '70s. [laughs]

INTERVIEWER: How did your success with the *Magic Mushroom Grower's Guide* steamroll into a career?

TERENCE: As the new age got going, say '80, '81, '82, I just found it incredibly irritating, and I was busy consulting and staying home and I also had small children, but I just thought it was such a bunch of crap.

INTERVIEWER: Talking about crystals and such?

TERENCE: Yeah, the crystal, aura, past life, channeling business, and I said, you know, why don't these people check out drugs? What's the matter with them, my god? And finally someone persuaded me to say that in a public situation, and it's been constant ever since.

Terence had farmed mushrooms until 1986, when he quit after an LSD-synthesizing friend was caught. "They fucked him so terrifyingly that I saw I couldn't do this anymore," he told *Wired* in 1999. After that, his main source of income became talks and tapes of talks. In 1984, Sound Photosynthesis had released a nine-hour, fourteen-minute "talking book" in which he examined the experiment at La Chorrera, and in 1985, he and Kathleen had founded Botanical Dimensions, an ethnobotany-dedicated nonprofit organization that included a garden on the Big Island of Hawaii. After he stopped farming mushrooms, he and his family moved to Hawaii and lived there in 1986 and some of 1987 before returning to California. By the late 1980s, Terence was speaking to audiences of sometimes around two thousand people. Publishers became "suddenly interested" in his work, he wrote in the preface to *True Hallucinations*.

8. BOOKS AND DIVORCE

In *Food of the Gods* (1992), his first non-co-written book—and first from a large publisher—Terence argued, via his Stoned Ape theory, that psilocybin-containing mushrooms caused the human brain-size to triple. He wanted to title the book—in which he recast Eve, portrayed in the Adam and Eve myth as easily tricked and deserving punishment, as brave, wise, and inspirational—*Why Eve Was Right: Plant, Drugs, and History*, but his publisher said no. "You learn your place in the hierarchy of being when you work with Bantam Books," he said on February 7, 1992, ten days before the book was published, and the audience laughed. "But, seriously, this is my best shot at making a rational argument—heh, sort of—based on archaeology, history, and so forth for the importance of psychedelics."

In the 313-page book, his longest, Terence also, in a part titled "Hell," told the histories of sugar, coffee, tea, chocolate, opium, tobacco, heroin, cocaine, and TV, showing bleak connections between sugar ("the world's least discussed and most widespread addiction") and slavery, the CIA and heroin, and the CIA and cocaine. The book's other three parts—"Paradise," "Paradise Lost," "Paradise Regained"—focused on "hallucinogens," as he called psychedelics in this book, whose last chapter included eight pages on DMT and a ten-item list—"A Modest Proposal"—that suggested cannabis be legalized and, with alcohol and tobacco, taxed 200 percent. "Since I feel pretty much among friends and fringies here, it doesn't trouble me to confess that my book *Food of the Gods* I really conceived of as a kind of intellectual Trojan horse," he said in a talk soon after it was published. Containing a bibliography, footnotes, and "citations of impossible-to-find books," the book seemed to be—and was—a scientific study. Another function, though, of this presentation was to "calm academic anthropologists" who out of the "staid, rational discourse" would find "self-transforming elves from hyperspace with their own agenda."

Terence's second book, published three months later, was less Trojan horse–like. Its characteristically long subtitle ("Speculations on Psychedelic Mushrooms, the Amazon, Virtual Reality, UFOs, Evolution, Shamanism, the Rebirth of the Goddess, and the End of History") accurately stated its contents. Its title—*The Archaic Revival*—referred to his idea that we should look back in time for help and solutions like the medieval world did in the Renaissance when they revived Greek and Roman ideas, except since our problem was worse, we should look back further, to before agriculture and civilization. The book collected six interviews, four transcribed talks, and seven essays, including "Among *Ayahuasqueros*," a "reflective diary" of Terence's trip with Kathleen, whom he described in *Food of the Gods* as "the best possible companion, colleague, and muse," to Peru in spring 1976, seven months before their marriage.

Sixteen years after that trip, in 1992, the year Terence published four books—the two mentioned, the limited-edition *Synesthesia*, and a collection of trialogues—they divorced.

9. *TRUE HALLUCINATIONS*

With his third non-co-written book—a poignant, sometimes zany, scene-based memoir—Terence, at age forty-six, in 1993, externalized the version of the story of his life that most people now know. *True Hallucinations* was an updated, print version of the talking book released in 1984 that had the same title. Changes included sentence-level edits, the excision of two UFO-focused chapters, and the addition of an epilogue, in which he shared that his marriage to Kathleen, despite their children and "efforts to be decent people," seemed to be ending—that the presence of the Logos, the teaching voice of the mushroom, had "done nothing to mitigate or ward off the ordinary vicissitudes of life."

Terence called *True Hallucinations* "the easy-to-read narrative anecdotal version" of *The Invisible Landscape*. The twenty-chapter, lightly footnoted book was centered around what happened at La Chorrera but also examined temporal mirages, Witoto history, avoiding "non-freaks," replacing "the ordinary anticipation of the future" with a Zen-like appreciation of the overall pattern, understanding sand dunes as lower-dimensional templates of wind, chronons, DNA, extraterrestrial life, his childhood, his career, and his family. Terence wrote cinematically and in a more exuberant, uninhibited prose than in his other, less personal books. He quoted his and Dennis's journals from when they were twenty-four and twenty. He wrote of "the every-colored stars," of "imagining what one *can* imagine."

He described what he felt as a twenty-four-year-old in 1971 smoking a joint on the Putumayo River—"on the edge of war-bloated, mad America," away from his mom's death months earlier and the loss of all his books and art a year earlier—on his way to La Chorrera with his brother and friends to find an obscure psychedelic drug: "The flow of smoke, the flow of water, and of time. 'All flows,' said a beloved Greek. Heraclitus was called the crying philosopher, as if he spoke in desperation. But, why crying? I love what he says—it does not make me cry. Rather than interpret *pante rhea* as 'nothing lasts,' I had always considered it a Western expression of the idea of Tao. And here we were, going with the Putumayo's flow."

10. FIRE AND CANCER

The year *True Hallucinations* was published, a year after his divorce, Terence began building his own house in Kona, Hawaii. "The first stop on the psychedelic trip is the library," he said in 1994 in Sherman, New York. In 1995, he created his website. "I spent all summer learning modeling and three-dimensional animation programs from my son because I want to animate," he said in Chicago in 1997. His talks evolved in the mid-to-late 1990s, including more on the internet, AI, nanotechnology, and computers while continuing to ponder old themes. "In the course of taking psychedelics and looking at my life and other people's lives and narrative, I think that the secret of—I don't want to say anything as pretentious as transcendence or enlightenment— but the secret of taking hold of one's destiny is to understand that one is a character," he said in San Francisco in December 1998. Psychedelics, he said in the same talk, spread alienation: "But what they alienate us from is preposterous, Earth-murdering, sexist, consumerist, shallow, trivial, inane, insane, and dangerous." In a two-titled talk—"Psychedelics in the Age of Intelligent Machines" and "Shamans Among the Machines"—in Seattle in April 1999, he discussed the "drug-like nature of the future," how drugs and computers are both "function-specific arrangements of matter," and the possibility of redeeming "the horror of history" by externalizing the soul into a "galaxy-roving vehicle."

At home three and a half weeks later, on May 22, 1999, he had a brain seizure and collapsed. A CAT scan showed a tumor in his right frontal cortex. He had glioblastoma multiforme, a rare form of brain cancer. From June 6, 1999, to April 3, 2000, ten updates were posted on his condition—written by himself; his brother; his editor on two of his books; and his girlfriend, whom he'd met a year earlier—on his website. "Generally my spirits are high and my life is certainly very interesting and more emotionally rich than before," he wrote on June 25, three weeks after undergoing Gamma Knife surgery. He was mostly in Honolulu for treatments, but his goal was to return every two weekends or so to his "secret rebel base on the Big Island"—the house he'd finally, a year earlier, completed.

Described as "a modernist origami structure topped with a massive antenna dish and a small astronomy dome" in a profile of Terence published in *Wired* three weeks after he died, the house was irrigated with rainwater collected on a hill, powered by solar panels and a gas generator, and had Ethernet connections "everywhere, even out on the deck" but no phone lines. The dome was for a telescope Terence couldn't afford. In the study, fourteen bookcases held his second library, which included rare first editions of alchemical texts and which, in 2007, while being stored by Esalen Institute, which planned to make it available to the public, would also, like his first, destruct in flames, this time not from wildfires but a fire beginning in a Quiznos. Around the house grew patches of white-and-purple-flowered *Salvia divinorum* and thick hanging vines of *Banisteriopsis caapi* with its pairs of opposing leaves.

"I'll try to be around and about," said Terence at a conference on the influence of psychedelics on artists held in Kona in part due to his failing health, seven months before he died. "But if I'm not, then you know that I'm behind your eyelids, and I'll meet you there."

EPILOGUE

When Terence died on April 3, 2000, at age fifty-three, his belongings included art, books, and an insect collection. In 2008, a year after his books were destroyed, his daughter, Klea, creatively preserved his insect collection in *The Butterfly Hunter*—a large, hardcover, olive-green book featuring photographs of 122 insects collected by Terence between 1969 and 1972. The butterflies, moths, and beetles were photographed with the magazine ads, newspaper articles, and typewritten manuscript pages in which Terence had wrapped them. Each photo was an arrangement, and each page was a part of a narrative. "The years of 1969 to 1972 were deeply formative for him; he had left home and childhood behind, but did not yet have a family or a public persona," wrote Klea in the book's introduction. "He was deciding who he would be."

I've told you about McKenna's worldview and life. Now I'll focus on psychedelics, which McKenna advocated for shamanic exploration, "personal growth work," and as "a force that forces us to grow up and clean up." To do this, I will first share my history with drugs. Before I was interested in psychedelics, I was interested in drugs.

MY DRUG HISTORY

My parents were born in Taiwan. They married on April 28, 1976, when my dad was twenty-eight and my mom was twenty-three, before coming to the United States that year (Dad) and the next (Mom), the only ones from their families of nine siblings combined to leave the island country. My dad borrowed money from my mom's dad for his plane ticket. In upstate New York, my mom waitressed and my dad earned a master's degree and doctorate in physics from the University of Rochester. My dad was thirty-five, my mom thirty, and my brother six when I was born on July 2, 1983, in Alexandria, Virginia. Two and a half years later, we moved to Florida, where we lived in three houses of increasing size in suburbs near Orlando called Apopka, Winter Springs, and Oviedo. My dad taught physics at the University of Central Florida and founded four medical laser companies while my mom raised my brother and me and helped my dad with his businesses—doing almost full-time work, including all the paperwork—and maintained our finances and household, which included Binky and Tabby, our toy poodles. My brother left for college in Philadelphia when I was eleven, and when I was eighteen, in 2001, I went to New York City, where I attended New York University, majoring in "undecided." I encountered no drugs in my first twenty-five years, except:

- Antibiotics for a fever when I was two or three and later for ear infections.

- Tylenol Cold, Tylenol Flu, Advil, and other store-bought drugs.

- Ten to fifteen vaccine shots containing glyphosate and other pesticides, thimerosal and other preservatives, and aluminum and other adjuvants.

- Thirty-plus injected, rubbed, and oral doses of benzodiazepines, opiates, and antibiotics from dentists and orthodontists.

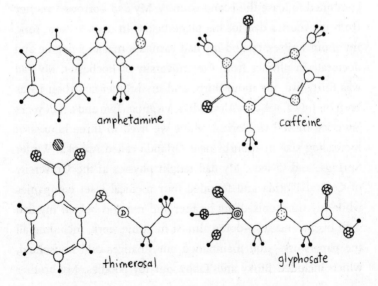

amphetamine

caffeine

thimerosal

glyphosate

- Nicotine, β-carbolines, pesticides, and additives from a cigarette in middle school.

- Cannabis once in high school.

- Morphine and other opiates fifteen to twenty-five times in hospitals in high school, when my right lung spontaneously collapsed three times.

- Ten or so Percocet (left over from twelfth-grade lung surgery) in college.

- Alcohol with little or no enjoyment twenty to thirty times.

- St. John's Wort, 5-HTP, and other legal mood-enhancers, which I dabbled in hopefully six to ten times, with disappointing results.

- Thousands of types of pesticides, antibiotics, hormones, chlorides and fluorides, artificial flavors and colors, and stray pharmaceuticals in food, water, lotions, soaps, shampoos, conditioners, and swimming pools.

- Caffeine from soda, coffee, and tea most days since middle school.

Except after caffeine, when for up to two hours, one to three times a day, I'd feel motivated and energized and happier, my experience of the world through my body—my felt presence of immediate experience—from 1983 to 2009 was, for reasons examined throughout this book, mostly one of frustratingly vague nausea, amoeboid posture, itchy skin, stuffed-up sinuses, multi-cold-sored lips and gums and throat, pain-threatening eyeball discomfort, debilitating headaches and stomachaches, worryingly long nosebleeds, uneasy eye movements, dysphoria, dyspnea, insomnia, bloatedness, and sluggishness.

Still, as a small child, I was very energetic. My mom called me hyperactive. I climbed things, ran around, felt excited. I easily smiled and laughed, sometimes for no reason. But in middle school most of that went away as I began to feel more often sickly, anxious, tired, awkward, self-conscious, and uncomfortable.

◎

D.A.R.E.

At Red Bug Elementary School, 1989 to 1994, ages six to ten, my dominant source of information regarding "drugs" was probably the Drug Abuse Resistance Education program. D.A.R.E., which manifested in school with police officers coming in to talk to us and on TV, billboards, and cars as commercials, advertisements, and stickers, "dared" children "to resist drugs and violence." My main memory of D.A.R.E. is of not understanding why resisting drugs was daring. The natural state of many of my classmates seemed to be low-level, casual violence—in the form of randomly punching and elbowing, or "bowing," as it was called, one another—so I understood how violence, which I disliked, partly because I was small and frail, was something some children would need to resist. But it seemed obviously riskier and braver—more daring—to try, instead of, like seemingly everyone, resist, drugs. The word "resist" in combination with the government's War on Drugs's motto "Just Say No" confused me because these messages seemed to assume I would occasionally, or at least once, be aggressively offered free drugs, a scenario I felt didn't make sense and would probably never happen.

D.A.R.E.'s psychology also confused me in terms of its logo, which was the acronym seemingly spray-painted—in a slanted, all-capital, bloodred graffito—against a solid black or white background. The design conveyed menace and anarchy, things that obviously, it seemed to me, encouraged drug use, violence, and other illegal behavior. My elementary-school mind, beginning in its unsuspecting way, in the long psychedelic trip of childhood, to discern deception in the world, sensed it was somehow unsound for D.A.R.E. to try to offer us what it thought we would, later in our lives, want from drugs—rebellion, disorder, chaos—as part of its strategy to keep us away from drugs.

But I didn't think about it much. In elementary school I didn't encounter "drugs." The word remained undifferentiated, referring to a single, bad substance I'd never seen.

GEMSTONE III

In middle school, 1994 to 1997, ages eleven, twelve, and thirteen, I continued encountering no drugs. In the minutes between classes, we played quick games of Magic: The Gathering, except my best friend at the time, Ryan, who wasn't allowed to have Magic cards because his Christian mom felt they were "evil." In fall 1995, some of us began playing a multiplayer text-based online role-playing game that had become available on AOL. Four or five classmates had already been playing it heavily for weeks, it seemed, when I learned about GemStone III, which, because it involved fantasy figures like orcs and sorcerers, Ryan also wasn't allowed to play.

Soon, I was playing GemStone III—a game in which I could type "east" to move my character, a dark elf wizard I'd named Esperath Wraithling, to a new location, which I "saw" by reading sentences describing his new surroundings—around six hours on school days and more on weekends. Normally, I didn't feel awake until third or fourth period; now I was waking early to play an unbeatable game set on a two-mooned planet called Elanthia for an hour or more, lucid and focused, before school. My friends and I began calling one another "addicts" derogatorily and defensively and understandingly. It became shameful to play too much, to spend so many hours engaged in a graphics-less, nonphysical activity. Anyone could type "find [name of character]" to learn if whomever was in the game—which cost something like $20 a month—so, except by creating a new character, it was impossible to hide how much we played. Most of us never saw one another on Elanthia; we did things alone or interacted with others—mostly adults, it seemed—across America who'd begun playing as early as 1990. When we met at Red Bug Lake Park to play basketball, we ended up betting GemStone III possessions on games of H-O-R-S-E or single, half-court shots before returning excitedly, after hours of abstinence, to our computers to be in a language-world that, at its peak, occupied around 2,500 humans simultaneously. We derived enjoyment and satisfaction through social interaction (like in an advanced chat room), by exploring Elanthia (like in a fractionally higher-dimensional novel), by amassing belongings (amulets, weapons), and by discerning numbers increase in a recorded, public manner.

At the peak, around ten children at Tuskawilla Middle School, that I was aware of, were "addicted," as we continued to call one another accusingly and sympathetically, with varying amounts of amused humor, which remained possible because there were so many of us, giving the reality of Elanthia some legitimacy. I was surprised to see some of us succumb this hard to a game of spells and kobolds and empaths—a friend who usually focused busily on extracurricular activities that colleges liked to see on application forms, at least two football players. Our time-consuming, antisocial behavior troubled some of our parents, but not others', and the children of the latter seemed to become the most obsessed. One classmate, named Brad, playing probably nine or ten hours a school day, rapidly advanced to level 80-something, becoming one of the most powerful characters in the history of the game, and ended up marrying someone in real life that he met on Elanthia.

I think my main character (I also had a halfling wizard and other characters) was level 28 when, after two years, around the beginning of high school, I stopped playing GemStone III.

PUNK MUSIC

In high school, 1997 to 2001, when I was fourteen, fifteen, sixteen, and seventeen, my interests included playing piano, playing drums at home and in Lake Howell High School's concert and marching bands, playing computer games with graphics, and listening to punk music. I encountered no drugs in the first three activities. The fourth, which I enjoyed almost exclusively alone, sometimes mentioned drugs and is also worth examining due to its influence on my worldview. I learned of punk music in middle school when (1) someone in GemStone III said I should listen to Operation Ivy and (2) in a record store I recognized the Descendents from one of my brother's T-shirts and bought their 1991 compilation album *Somery*. In high school, I often listened to punk music as my only activity (before and after school, between classes through earphones, in my car, in bed before sleep), focusing on the lyrics, vocals, guitars, bass, or drums. Using Napster, which was active from June 1999 to July 2001, I downloaded thousands of songs.

Punk music primed me for Terence McKenna's ideas, many of which I first encountered in lyrics and liner notes in simpler, angrier, catchier, more emotional, less contextualized form. The bands I listened to rarely sang about paranormal, extradimensional, or mystical topics; didn't seem obsessed with psychedelics; and sparingly referenced deep time, but punk music and McKenna overlapped in many other ways. Both disapproved of materialism and consumerism and organized religion, advocated liberal and humanist and DIY ideas, viewed knowledge as power and trusted books, and distrusted and criticized the media, governments, corporations, textbooks, TV, and mainstream culture. They comfortably occupied antiestablishmentarianist, esoteric but not unpopular, deliberately independent positions in music and philosophy, with McKenna remaining outside academia and punk bands releasing albums through labels, like Asian Man Records and No Idea Records, started and owned by friends.

Before "punk music," a broad term I'll stop using now to focus on specific bands, I didn't consider why every morning at school I put my right hand on my chest and slowly recited allegiance to the United States flag in unison with my classmates. Now one of my favorite bands, the Broadways, had a song that began "Do you remember the first thing you had to memorize? / Was it the Pledge of Allegiance? / A five-year-old stands for a flag / that killed off all the real Americans."

I'd previously never encountered sentences like these, which I began absorbing daily from sung and screamed lyrics by almost all males in their twenties. The Broadways, who seemed to be four undergraduate students in Chicago, taught me, in their albums *Broken Star* (1998) and *Broken Van* (2000), to seek wisdom and sanity from nature, to question "progress" and technology, and to pay attention—not to celebrities and advertisements but to the poor and homeless and indigenous and underprivileged. They suggested that working 9 to 5, then watching TV from 6 to 10, wasn't good. My favorite song by them began "All down the streets the signs read / cheaper and better technology / this capitalist vision is my nightmare / put up a sign in my face / what the fuck happened to this place? / I think we made a wrong turn / look at the ugly concrete" and ended "And I wonder if this crazy world / thinks I'm the one who's crazy / What if I'm the one who's crazy? (×4) / I'm not crazy just frustrated."

Another band that consistently and provocatively moved me was Choking Victim, whose songs excerpted talks by the political scientist Michael Parenti. "Born to die and you get / to sit and watch your TV set / believe the lies before your eyes, credit cards and apple pies / Fifty stars to blind your eyes, thirteen stripes to hypnotize / free thought is gone / you'll never see you're just a pawn," began their three-minute, twenty-seven-second song "Born to Die," which used the same chord progression as "Wild Thing" and was from their *Squatta's Paradise* EP, which was released in 1996, the same year as Adderall. In "Fuck America," from their 1999 album *No Gods/No Managers*, Stza, the New York City band's vocalist and guitarist, sang, "McDonald's will bloom as the major competition / Between Jesus and the devil for this country's religion."

Atom and His Package—one person with a drum machine—had an upbeat, catchy, gleeful song praising Rob Halford, the singer of Judas Priest, a heavy metal band, for coming out as gay. In the song's chorus, Adam Goren sang that he wanted to be a homosexual. Since elementary school, probably 70 to 90 percent of my classmates and maybe a third to half my teachers had blithely used the concept of homosexuality in a derogatory manner, calling people or things "gay" as a synonym for "bad." I had done this also but then had felt self-conscious and stopped, somehow realizing it didn't make sense and was hurtful and mindless. I'd felt alone in my change. Hearing "Hats Off to Halford," a song my peers would call "gay" and be unable to enjoy, I was touched and startled, feeling more and less alone—more because I had no one to share the song with, less because the song indicated people existed who felt similarly as me.

The message from these bands regarding "drugs" varied, but all seemed to view them differently than on TV and at school. Propagandhi, whose albums included spoken word by Noam Chomsky, had members who outspokenly used no drugs. NOFX's song "Drugs Are Good" observed that when you use drugs people think you're cool. Jeff Ott, singer of Fifteen, was born in 1970 to a drug-addicted teenager as the result of a gang rape and used drugs intravenously from when he was fifteen to around twenty-four. In "War on Drugs," a song on Fifteen's 1999 album *Lucky*, Ott sang that the war's enemies were young black men, Mexicans, poor whites, and homeless people. He sang that his enemies were not heroin junkies, speed freaks, or skid row alcoholics and that his enemy did not sleep on the street. In "My Congressman," he shared how to clean a syringe with bleach and argued against politicians who said legalizing clean-needle exchanges would be "sending the wrong message" by pointing out that the message of magazines, TV, billboards, and stores was to buy cigarettes and alcohol.

These bands deromanticized and, more than other sources I'd encountered, differentiated "drugs" for me. They connected drugs to the CIA, Hollywood, racism, despair, mindlessness, being a victim of a larger system, and other topics that made drugs seem more complicated than before. Unlike MTV, most movies, programs like D.A.R.E., and authority figures like the president, these bands, which largely constituted my "friends" in high school, did not make drugs seem especially mysterious, interestingly taboo, extreme, dangerous, desirable, or transgressive.

LITERATURE

In college, from 2001 to 2005, I continued listening to the bands I did in high school but began preferring lyrics about feeling bad socially, romantically, and especially for "no concrete reason," as I liked to think of it. I sought and collected and prized lyrics that directly expressed or examined social anxiety, low self-esteem, depression, loneliness, disappointment, disillusionment, and resignation in a personal, non-sociological, apolitical manner. Some bands from high school had formed new bands that lyrically mirrored my preference change—Propagandhi's bassist had formed the Weakerthans, whose lyrics poetically explored meek desperation and controlled longing; members of the Broadways were now in the Lawrence Arms, and they still sang about homeless people but added more on unrequited feelings and having low motivation in life. "Sixty watts, brighter than my future; an empty forty, fuller than my life," sang Jim Marburger in "Less Than Nothing," a song by a band called I Hate Myself.

I wanted elaboration—paragraphs, scenes, stories, characters, worlds—and I found it in literature, which I had begun reading in high school after watching *Fight Club* and, identifying with its characters' alienation and unhappiness, going to Chuck Palahniuk's website and finding, from his recommendations, Kurt Vonnegut, Don DeLillo, and Amy Hempel. I bought

Hempel's out-of-print collections *Reasons to Live* (1985) and *At the Gates of the Animal Kingdom* (1990) off eBay and, in my first year of college, read her stories repeatedly, as if they were songs. From Hempel, I found Raymond Carver, Mary Robison, Frederick Barthelme, and others. I became especially interested in short stories—the gamely, brazenly purified novels of them, their almost memorizable arcs and complex epiphanies and valuable rereadability, with many stories, like those by Lorrie Moore and Lydia Davis and Joy Williams, startling and moving and transporting me as much on the first reading as the third. I read and reread *The Book of Disquiet*, a book of fragments by Fernando Pessoa (1888–1935), published in Portuguese in 1982 and English in 1991. "Tedium is not the disease of being bored because there's nothing to do, but the more serious disease of feeling that there's nothing worth doing," wrote Pessoa. In a self-profile published in *The Stranger* in 2010, I described myself during this time, in college, as "lonely and friendless but mutedly excited about autobiographical narratives featuring characters with low serotonin."

Those—and other—writers affected and delighted me with their intimate, detached, amusing, wry, melancholic, quietly desperate, non-melodramatic, calming, loneliness-reducing portrayals of mundane, realistic worlds, often from outsider perspectives. "I would never be part of anything," wrote Jean Rhys (1890–1979), who I discovered by Googling variations of "depressing lonely novel" at night in New York University's library, in her unfinished, posthumous autobiography. "I would never really belong anywhere, and I knew it, and all my life would be the same, trying to belong, and failing. Always something would go wrong. I am a stranger and I always will be, and after all I didn't really care."

Drugs, in the form of alcohol, featured in many of my favorite novels, like *Chilly Scenes of Winter* by Ann Beattie and *The Easter Parade* by Richard Yates, both from 1976, but never became the main theme. In Rhys's *Good Morning, Midnight* (1939), Sasha Jensen, an Englishwoman living alone in Paris in 1937, drank heavily and used Luminal, a product created by Bayer in 1912 that contained phenobarbital, seemingly nightly—"I am not sad as I go upstairs, not sad, not happy, not regretful, not thinking of anything much. Except that I see very clearly in my head the tube of luminal and the bottle of whisky." In *Anagrams* (1986) by Lorrie Moore, a character told the reader that sedatives helped one "adjust to death better." Psychedelics never featured and were rarely mentioned in my favorite books. The term "drugs" often wasn't differentiated, like in "Willing," Moore's 1990 story about an actress living in a hotel room that was "L-shaped, like a life veering off suddenly to become something else" in Chicago:

> She would try then not to think too strenuously about her *whole life*. She would try to live life one day at a time, like an alcoholic—drink, don't drink, drink. Perhaps she should take drugs.

This partially joke-like view of "drugs," as a symbol for giving up on or starting a new kind of life, was the one I embodied most during college, when I was alone most of the time, reading and writing. I graduated in 2005 with a degree in journalism and minors in creative writing and psychology. In 2006, 2007, and 2008, I published four books and rarely thought about drugs—except caffeine, which I strategically used every day and thought about, on some level, constantly.

ADDERALL AND METHADONE

In 2009, when I was twenty-six, after reading about it for months online, including in an essay in the fall 2008 issue of *n+1* magazine called "Kickstart My Heart," I began wanting Adderall, a drug made by Shire Pharmaceuticals that contained amphetamine, colloidal silicon dioxide, compressible sugar, cornstarch, magnesium stearate, microcrystalline cellulose, saccharin sodium, and FD&C Blue #1, an 87-atom compound, or FD&C Yellow #6, a 39-atom compound. In March, a friend in Seattle mailed me three Adderall. The effects surprised me, seeming much more powerful than I'd anticipated. Using only 5 or 10 milligrams at a time, it made me feel like a hard-working, fast-moving, social, contented robot. It provided mental acuity, motivation, and improved mood for hours in which I existed as another person who was less grumpy and immobile and inhibited.

In April, I bought something like sixty 20-milligram Adderall from my then girlfriend Sarah's friend. In July, a different friend of Sarah's injured herself and received methadone, which she gave to Sarah, and which Sarah and I enjoyed around once a week, walking around SoHo and the Lower East Side in twilight, eating in restaurants, seeing movies, sleeping. It lasted much longer than Adderall, sometimes into the next afternoon, providing pleasurable calmness and a subtle, ancient-seeming, fuzzy sensation of not being worried about anything. A search of "methadone" in my Gmail shows that Sarah and I were excited that summer about opiates and other drugs, that we discussed how to get more drugs, but our relationship ended in November.

Compared to Adderall and methadone, caffeine—which had previously impressed me often—seemed weak and unsatisfying, its effects so comparatively brief that it now usually just caused me to feel distractingly and discouragingly aware that, within minutes, I'd feel zombielike and unenthused again. After Adderall and methadone, drugs that gifted me levels of energy and collectedness I'd never felt before, I realized I'd underestimated the strength and usefulness of drugs, partly because I'd suspected people of faking how powerful they were and partly because of all the inaccurate drug information I'd absorbed since grade school.

"RECOVERY"

In spring 2010, I began using "drugs" in a staggered but increasingly regular manner; the word differentiated to tens of words, each indicating a drug or category of drug that I wanted to try. I excitedly viewed drugs as tools I could use to significantly change my underlying experience of life—how I felt while I wrote, talked to people, went to parties, watched movies, read books, exercised, typed emails, browsed websites, gave readings. Aware that millions of children and adults used Adderall, methadone, and other, presumably as-powerful drugs daily for years and even decades, I felt encouraged to incorporate more drugs into my life. Aware that most people ate terrible food that damaged their bodies more, I estimated, than drugs would damage mine—and that, unfortunately, food provided only seconds of an elusive, emotionless pleasure, not minutes to hours of productivity and emotional euphoria and intimacy with one's peers—I was encouraged to use more drugs and also to eat healthier food, choices that I felt benefited both myself and others. People interacting with a drugged, nourished me encountered a pleasanter, less dismaying, often more attentive person. I was grateful and often giddy for drugs. Used consciously in a relevant, real-life game, amphetamines and benzodiazepines and opiates and MDMA—and

other, stranger drugs, like LSD and psilocybin, which I began trying that summer—made my life more vivid, poignant, peopled,
exciting, and interconnected.

But drugs also made my life bleaker, emptier, scarier, and
more troubling. Always aware of the reality of tolerance—that
I needed to use more each time to achieve the same effect and
so was still, with drugs, required to endure uncomfortable and
interminable hours and days—I was always, on some level, worried about my situation. I entered more social situations and
communicated more fulfillingly with drugs than without, but I
also spent more consecutive hours alone in my room wishing a
"sleep machine" existed that I could use, by pushing a button, to
instantly fall asleep. I became accustomed to not being in a social
situation unless also on a drug. Soon, I didn't want to do anything, even solitary activities, unless I was on at least one drug
or, increasingly, two. It had once been a funny joke to want to be
on both Adderall and Xanax—an upper and a downer—but now
it became mundane and humorlessly "not a good sign." Sometimes, I wanted to refrain for a day or two or three—which I did
gradually less—so the drugs would work better when I restarted,
but I would easily convince myself why I should, in this par-
ticular instance, not refrain, citing any reason or combination
of reasons from "it will benefit me as an artist" to "I could die
at any moment" to "I should be extra-impulsive sometimes to
jostle and challenge my underprovoked brain and for variety." I
would sometimes not think anything, but just take more, aware
I was mindlessly giving in to what most of me wanted. Then I
would feel both troubled and dimly amused to have, again, either
rationalized myself into or just, after initial indecision, observed
myself using more drugs.

Despite viewing myself as in a committed, long-term process
to use less drugs, I found myself using gradually more in an

increasingly habitual, uncontrolled manner—a paradox I've con-
ceptualized in this book as my "recovery." I began to "recover"
from drugs in fall 2010. Some of the time, usually while on
drugs, I became convinced and even told people that I was actually becoming happier as I used more drugs—that somehow the
chemicals were doing something beneficial to my brain, maybe
causing cells to grow that, unlike the old ones, knew how to
be happy—but most of the time I knew my behavior was definitely and disturbingly leading to more anxiety and depression.
My "recovery" continued through 2011 and 2012, when sometimes I felt that maybe I would die soon, or eventually, from
drugs, low self-esteem, self-caused lovelessness, unstructured
days and nights, unexamined expectations I'd absorbed from
various sources in culture, a complicatedly uncomfortable experience of my body, not belonging to any group except myself,
living alone, an at least somewhat romanticized perspective on
all these things that would kill me, and a bleak worldview. Many
people had died from combinations of those things, and now I
would. It made sense and seemed normal. "There's a horribly
frightening little passage in Jung somewhere, where he says,
'The unconscious has a thousand ways to terminate a life that
has become meaningless,'" said McKenna, who I encountered
in the depths of my "recovery," in a talk in 1994. "Meaning you'll
step in front of a streetcar, or something." I imagine that's how
I could have died—in a manner seeming, even to myself, with
my level of consciousness being, most of the time, lower than
ever, accidental.

   In January 2013, I went to live with my parents (who'd moved
back to Taiwan in 2006 after thirty years in "beautiful country,"
as the United States is called in Mandarin) for around a month,
during which, viewing myself (in a disempowering manner that
was paradoxically helpful) as physically unable to obtain drugs—

because my Mandarin was bad, I feared social interaction as much as not having drugs, I had no friends in Taiwan, and I wasn't close to my relatives—my recovery began.

RECOVERY

In my parents' fifth-floor apartment in Taipei, I felt deep underground. Sometimes I felt, even more unexpectedly, "beneath" the substrate of concrete reality in some kind of dimensionally recessed state. At night, in bed, in my room that was comfortingly lit by lunar and municipal light through large windows, I felt scared. In the day, I tasted metal in my mouth. By my request, I received Xanax in the mail from a friend, but only once; otherwise I used only caffeine.

I returned to New York in February 2013 and restarted Adderall, Xanax, and other drugs in somewhat considerable amounts, including thirty-six- to forty-eight-hour, room-based, stimulant-centered binges, but much less than in 2012 and 2011. As my drug use decreased, my knowledge and use of psychedelics increased. In Taiwan, I'd read *True Hallucinations* and *The Brotherhood of the Screaming Abyss*, and now I ordered Terence and Dennis's earlier books and other books from psychedelia. With help from cannabis, psilocybin, the McKenna brothers, myself, my parents, and my history, including the inspiration and reasons to live I'd absorbed from punk music and literature, my "recovery" ended at the end of August—a month when I had a seminal psilocybin trip (examined in the next chapter) and, on a weeklong book tour in the UK with a fellow drug-enjoying friend, my last drug binge, as I considered it at the time but later recast, within an overall plan of decreasing usage, as *one of* my last binges.

The first eight months of 2013, I was both "recovering" and

recovering. In September, my recovery finally continued alone, without its bleak counterpart. I continued decreasing my use of amphetamines, benzos, and opiates (I'd stopped MDMA months earlier with ease because I'd felt aversion toward it since using it to discomforting excess in late 2010 and early 2011) and started smoking cannabis daily. I began to "regain control of my brain," as I thought of it and sometimes told people. After two or three months, with a kind of surprise that was itself surprising, I felt able to realistically envision a future that didn't just get worse, or stay the same, but would actually—almost mechanically—get better, or at least feel better, over weeks and months, as I recovered from years of dependences on various drugs. I comprehended how, just by abstaining from damaging behaviors I'd habitualized, life would gradually feel different—which would affect my thoughts and worldview—and the idea seemed pleasing and surreal.

On January 10, 2014, after using only cannabis for around a week, abstaining even from caffeine, I felt unexpectedly content and peaceful. I'd known I would feel better over time, but I was still, in my room that afternoon, surprised it was happening, that I had the power and opportunity to give myself a gradual, barely noticeable, never-ending psychedelic experience, without a peak or denouement, arcing across years instead of hours, going somewhere without coming back. My life, I sensed with some clarity, could slowly become vastly different. I wanted to remind my future self about this feeling, so I typed a paragraph, wrote it on paper, and taped the paper to my wall, then screenshotted the paragraph, emailed it to myself, and made it my phone's background. I didn't want to forget:

I was beginning to change—happier, more interested in things—this afternoon, I could feel. It's incremental change in one direction every day, because I'm recovering from 10–20 years caffeine, 4–7 years other drugs, etc.* So it will lead me somewhere new and unfamiliar. This is how I can get out of my life. This is how life can be exciting and interesting again. This is how my life, after 30 years, can slowly adventure into the unknown, instead of stalling here.

BRIEF ANALYSIS OF MY DRUG HISTORY

I began late, not starting non-caffeine drugs until twenty-six and psychedelics until twenty-seven. As a writer interested in describing my experience of the world through varied states of conscious-

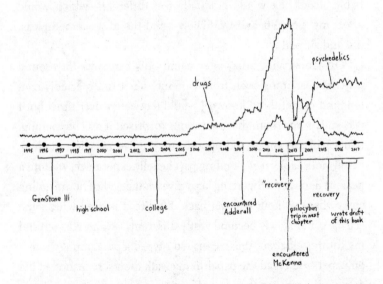

* I overestimated with "4–7"—I'd been using drugs in considerable amounts for around three-and-a-half years. With "etc." I referred to the culture I'd consumed, my thoughts and goals, and my malnourished, toxified, dysbiotic, inactive, understimulated body.

ness, my late start seems advantageous. I like to imagine that, instead of immediately using it habitually once I learned to enjoy it, I deliberately and wisely, with impressively delayed gratification, abstained (mostly) from cannabis until I was thirty, so that its effects, against the backdrop of three decades of non-stoned consciousness, would be more distinctive and powerful and so that, by then, I'd have a decade of practice in languaging experience. My drug history is also notable, besides my late start, for shifting almost completely from drugs to psychedelics—taking thirty-two years to attain a satisfyingly balanced, I feel, looking at my graph, arrangement.

DIFFERENCES BETWEEN PSYCHEDELICS AND DRUGS

The word "drugs" referred to one thing for most of my life, then to uppers and downers, then to stimulants and MDMA and benzodiazepines and opiates, and so on, but now I found it most useful, personally and in terms of this book, to differentiate the word to two main categories—drugs and psychedelics, which could specify to tryptamines (psilocybin, DMT, LSD), phenethylamines (mescaline, 2C-B), and others (THC, salvinorin A). One similarity between psychedelics and drugs is that we are always experiencing both, are always on fluctuating amounts of serotonin, DMT, GABA, adenosine, oxytocin, dopamine, opioids, cannabinoids, and hundreds of other compounds for which we've evolved receptors. The amounts we are on, and their ratios, determine, or at least strongly influence, our realities. "Life itself is a drug experience," said Dennis McKenna, who earned a PhD in botanical science in 1984 and has published around forty papers on psychedelics, in an interview in 1994. Seven differences:

1. Drugs are, on average, more habit-forming than psychedelics, which can also, like almost anything, be habitforming, but, unlike drugs, can also dissolve habits.

2. Drugs don't cause mystical experiences at safe doses; psychedelics do, as was shown in 1962 in the Good Friday Experiment in which graduate divinity students ingested psilocybin or a placebo. Eight of ten on psilocybin had mystical experiences, and in a study twenty-four years later on seven of the eight, all seven viewed their experience as "one of the high points of their spiritual life."

3. For me, drugs stopped feeling amazing after the first few times—and never felt profound—but psychedelics consistently feel both amazing and profound. The word "profound" had little meaning for me before psychedelics—before, among their other effects, I experienced reality so differently that, from the rare far vantage, I discerned the utter weirdness of normal existence.

4. Drugs don't seem to guarantee relief from boredom. Psychedelics I would immediately rate 10 on a 1–10 scale for boredom relief, even for the easily bored, because they seem to catalyze the imagination through stimulation, like some drugs, but also at least two other ways, bringing in emotion and the unconscious.

5. In fall 2014, while doing interviews for the German edition of *Taipei*—which I wrote during a period of increasing drug use, from early 2010 to late 2012, about a previous, overlapping period of increasing drug use, from

November 2009 to August 28, 2011—I was asked, after directing conversation there myself, about the difference between psychedelics and drugs. I said one difference was that drugs affected my energy levels, mood, focus, and other attributes—calmness, patience—that I experienced noticeable fluctuations in while sober, for example depending on how much I'd slept. Psychedelics seemed to affect aspects of consciousness that normally changed only slightly, if at all.

6. Another difference seemed to be that drugs increased my current levels by taking from the future. When the future arrived, I felt the lack of what I'd already used. Psychedelics, I told one or two journalists, didn't seem to take from the future. Months later, then, I noticed that if I smoked cannabis all day—and all day felt partly in a dream—then at night I didn't dream, and that when I abstained I dreamed vividly. I realized psychedelics, or at least cannabis, did seem to take from the future. Cannabis seemed to take something that was felt during sleep.

7. In early 2016, on Vimeo, I watched a 2015 talk by Kathleen Harrison in which she said psychedelics awakened compassion in her. I realized they did in me also, and that drugs did not. On Xanax around my parents, I've never felt almost overwhelmingly endeared by their behavior and perceived them as children, as I have on cannabis and LSD. Peaking on large doses of Adderall alone in my room, I've never sobbed while thinking fondly and lovingly about my parents, as I have on cannabis and psilocybin.

⊗

"I am not an advocate of drugs; I am an advocate of psychedel-ics," said Terence McKenna, who felt it was "too early for a sci-ence" regarding the psychedelic experience. "What we need now are the diaries of explorers," he said in an interview in 1989. "We need many diaries of many explorers so we can begin to get a feel for the territory." In the next two chapters, I examine my and his experiences with the two compounds he promoted most—psilocybin and DMT.

PSILOCYBIN

On August 5, 2013, at around 12:50 A.M., in my fourth-floor apartment on 29th Street in Manhattan, I ate 2.5 grams of an unknown species of dried, psilocybin-containing mushroom. I ate over forty to fifty minutes, motivated partially out of boredom, nibbling absentmindedly while feeling, as I did those days, in 2013, less doomed than one or two years earlier, but only a little and not consistently. Sometimes I still felt "non-humorously fucked," as I thought with varying amounts of humor; this was my eighth and final month both "recovering" and recovering. I had no plans that night, except to eventually sleep.

Seated at my desk, part of me felt like the mushrooms wouldn't do anything. I hadn't had psilocybin in around two months, so had forgotten the strangeness and potency of its effects and reverted somewhat to my view of psychedelics prior to eating mushrooms three years earlier—that they probably weren't as intense as people claimed. People seemed to use the same words to describe food and naps and images and normal reality—amazing, profound, mind-blowing, unbelievable—as psychedelic experiences not, I'd realized over time, because they were lying, and not necessarily because they were being characteristically hyperbolic, but because the phenomenology of psychedelics was difficult "to English," as McKenna said in "In the Valley of Novelty" (1998), observing that psilocybin and DMT seemed to particularly affect "the language-forming portions of the brain," which resulted in "bizarre states of mind" because it was these portions that explained what was happening.

Psilocybin's initial, rumblingly stimulating effects prodded me from my near-catatonic state, gazing at things with slow eye movements and no distinct thoughts, a common status for me in 2013, into a healthier mode of detail-oriented, collegial behavior: I began packing my other 2.5 grams of mushrooms to mail to a friend, who was at Yaddo, to nurture her interest in psychedelics. My calm productivity continued as I emailed her a photo of the package and a block of phone-typed text, recommending she eat the mushrooms alone at night with no obligations the next day (which was my situation) and sharing a little about my mushroom experiences:

- I'd eaten mushrooms ten to fifteen times in the past three years.

- I'd rarely eaten them alone. I'd eaten them before a reading, before going to the American Museum of Natural History, before seeing movies in theaters, at social gatherings, and with friends in the city and elsewhere.

- Around five times I'd concluded, for minutes, that I'd died.

- The most I'd eaten at once was probably 3 or 4 grams. That night was the first time I'd weighed a dose.

- Whenever I ate more than maybe around 1.5 grams, the intensity and alienness of the effects re-amazed me, causing me to think, "How could I have forgotten this?"

After sending my email at 1:44 A.M., my room began to feel spaceship-like. In my liver, 36-atom molecules of psilocybin were breaking down into 31-atom molecules of psilocin, which were entering my brain, where they were interacting with serotonin and other receptors. I felt myself leaving Earth in an intimidatingly disquieting manner, like I was on a vessel I hadn't suspected to exist, departing a place I'd assumed was the only place.

FLOOR

Feeling exposed and distractedly physical on my chair, I moved to the floor, sitting cross-legged with palm-up hands on the sides of my knees to relax and center myself. I lowered my eyelids, ending visual input of the locked, artificially lit concrete box of my room, which was permeated by microwaves from my phone, computer, router, and other apartments. Instead of the usual placeless darkness, I was calmly surprised to gradually—over around twenty seconds, with a certain mental effort—find myself in an unfamiliar, off-sunny, un-gaudily shimmering expanse.

Focusing various distances and directions into my eyelids, I looked at this place. Its golden, slightly visceral appearance modulated subtly and rapidly. Sometimes I didn't seem to be in an alien sky, but an incomprehensibly advanced structure with busily morphing tiles on every surface.

Wanting to explore, I tried to hover directionally as a cursor-like perspective, but I couldn't seem to move. I realized I was still required to think while disembodied. Somewhat troublingly, I couldn't just exist and feel. I was like a baby here, unable to do anything. I acknowledged I might explore this place—the imagination—better with more psilocybin and a healthier mind and body.

I became aware of a dull attention from a presence in the distance and instinctively wanted to raise my eyelids—to regain the privacy I normally enjoyed in my room—but didn't, partly because it wouldn't make sense; I'd be acting like Tabby, my family's charmingly awkward toy poodle who would hide her head and seem to believe we couldn't see her because she couldn't see us. I defaulted to a waiting-based stasis, and we settled into what felt vaguely like a pre-social situation.

Except in ways that I quickly discerned were just me paranoidally imagining things, I had never encountered a seemingly independent abstraction like this. Part of me rationalized it as an electromagnetic burst elsewhere in the building—a giant TV turning on in a room on another floor, forty feet away, maybe—that I was abnormally detecting, due to reconfigured senses on psilocybin, and had partially interpreted as an entity in the imagination.

In *Heaven and Hell* (1956), published when he was sixty-one, Aldous Huxley wrote about how "the aid of a chemical—either mescaline or lysergic acid"—brought one to the "antipodes" of the mind, which like Earth in the mid-nineteenth century still had its "unmapped Borneos and Amazonian basins." Earth's antipodes had duck-billed platypi and marsupials. "And if you go to the antipodes of the self-conscious mind, you will encounter all sorts of creatures at least as odd as kangaroos," wrote Huxley. People, in his view, could not control these oddities; we could only visit "the mental equivalent of Australia" and "look around."

Before anything happened, the thing—already somewhat in the distance—drifted dirigibly away, seeming incurious in me in a way that made it seem realer. Its casual indifference gave its world a mundane, universe-like quality.

BED

I climbed on my bed and lay supine. As I pulled my childhood blanket over me with slow-moving, funny-feeling hands, it seemed disturbingly different than ever before. It felt frighteningly complicated, comprised of startlingly minuscule Lego blocks, which increasingly also formed the air and my bed and, in a slowly engulfing way, my body. I felt precariously maintained as a conscious being by the liquidly recombining, intershuffling, everywhere blocks. This briefly felt fun in an obscure, risky, claustrophobic, darkly zany way. Then I felt I was "sinking" in a way that seemed hazardous.

Soon I became convinced that something I didn't comprehend had malfunctioned—which made sense because things broke all the time—and that now I was stuck and unlocatable. I seemed secluded inside a mountain on a lifeless planet. Not in a mountain cave, or the solid mountain itself, but an X-Y-Z-T coordinate (with T being time) in the finished object of the universe that marked the inside of a mountain somewhere. To find me, others would need to "dig" from a higher dimension—something, I sensed, that wasn't done. I was "encased" where none would look. This was my life now. I was fucked.

After realizing all this began when I lay on my bed and stopped moving, I felt glad and relieved. I stood and shakily walked three steps to my sofa, where I sat.

SOFA

Holding a ringed binder of watercolor paper and a red crayon, ready to write or draw something, I sensed the pointlessness of recording information outside oneself, something I'd also sensed four days earlier after smoking a non-threshold dose of DMT. "Crayons," I wrote in words covering almost half the paper, surprising myself a little. The word seemed written to occupy an unsuspecting majority of me so that a smaller part of me could analyze the concept of note-taking in private.

Note-taking seemed misguided and neurotic. Experience was the only usable information—takable from existence in the universe—and it was recorded automatically. My life *was* notes, etched into the four-dimensional object of the universe. Or was that just my behavior? My thoughts and feelings left no trace here; they went into books and then other minds.

I became distractedly hyper-focused on the screen-like nature of my vision. My face was so near the screen of my life that it was all I could see. This was normal, I reminded myself. I saw my crayon-grasping hand and other, lower-resolution things, like my wooden floor.

"Watching this," I wrote below "Crayons" in smaller letters.

I began to feel like I was an alien experiencing the life of a human named Tao Lin. I seemed to have my own life elsewhere but was currently "reading" the higher-dimensional book of Tao Lin. Once he died, I would return to my real life. I could sense my family—a partner and two children, it seemed—desiring my return in a moderate, healthy, appreciated manner. "I'll be there soon, I just have to do this thing," I thought without dread or despair, referring to Tao Lin's life, which I sensed I was living, was enduring and enjoying, for financial reasons. Pleased that life apparently involved much more than I previously thought, I felt eager yet patient to return to my world. All I knew now was Tao Lin, but soon I would complete my job and, with the satisfaction of a long-term task accomplished, return to my life wiser and more financially secure. I sensed maybe I was here not for money but to gather information. To collect data on humans. I reviewed my notes, to which I'd at some point added a third line:

Crayons
Watching this
i'll be there soon

Taking notes seemed pointless. I knew I'd already realized this. I felt calm and restless. I'd learned my alien heritage, ascertained and affirmed my situation as an extraterrestrial being, and communicated warmly with my real family. I was ready to move on to other topics.

BED AGAIN

I returned to my bed, where instead of lying supine, which could invoke Lego ontology, I sat cross-legged and forgot I was an alien. I thought about my life and sobbed, realizing I was finally going to end years of decreasingly enjoyable drug use. I'd "realized" this before but never this confidently, this lucidly. It felt actualized already. I cried thinking about how I was going to distance myself from the writing world and Twitter and Facebook and all culture except books and maybe movies and live alone in a rural area and publish a book about it or never publish another book but just disappear and maybe much later emerge messianically with a book or just never reemerge. I felt surprisingly able to decide what to do in terms of years and decades instead of hours and days, as if the decisions were literary.

I cried at what was happening.

My plan changed sometimes. I felt I would contentedly settle into a long-term relationship—countering my history of relationships lasting around a year each—and use my free time to leisurely research and carefully explore the mystery. I was, uncharacteristically, convinced, for minutes, that I would have children.

At 3:08 A.M., physically uncomfortable and becoming seemingly depressed, unsure if the effects were still intensifying and not wanting to be in a tensely unhappy mood, I used half a Xanax bar, which contained alprazolam, cellulose, cornstarch, docusate sodium, lactose, magnesium stearate, silicon dioxide, and sodium benzoate.

From 3:37 A.M. to 3:43 A.M., sitting on my bed sobbing, I tweeted "337," "339," "340," "Resting," "Resting on 340," "Then 341," "I'm crying," and "343" from my iPhone. I felt sometimes outside time, like time was a planet whose waves I floated on in a boat, beneath the stars of other worlds. Time was keeping me here, conscious.

At 3:46 A.M., I tweeted "I'm leaving behind all this lit game shit. I'm laughing. I dunno what I'm leaving behind in specific terms but I'm cutting it all off bye" from my MacBook. *Taipei* had been published two months earlier. On drugs at the release party, seated, I'd signed books seemingly the entire time for a line of people who kept coming, including ones who gifted me half-filled bottles of drugs that I accepted with private chagrin.

I noticed through bleary eyes, with some confusion, that the boxes on the screen didn't conceal their contents. Words and sentences were inside boxes, but I could see and change them, looking down into the lower dimension of the screen. This cross-dimensional access felt poignant and revelatory. I suddenly felt it didn't matter how I released information—emails, texts, tweets, even thoughts. My thoughts seemed public and findable in a higher dimension whose existence made life as relatively insignificant as the contents of a book. My tears felt dense and complex as blood. I encouraged my crying, sometimes viewing it as an uncommon, beneficial exercise. The next hour and a half included these atypical behaviors:

- With my hands covering my face, I forgot I could move my hands off my face, then moved them off my face and wondered why they weren't attached to my face.

- I texted and/or called four friends. Usually, I did not call anyone and rarely initiated texting, especially at around 5:00 A.M. "Listen: an alien was in me," I texted Gian, the only friend to respond until hours later. "It was using my body to figure out this terrain!" An alien, I said, was using me to "scope out this place," to learn about "this thing we've got set up: family." Gian, who I knew used psilocybin to treat his cluster headaches, responded, "You don't think they have families?" I answered, "I'm laughing / No they do / Of course they do / I respect that," called him, and we talked for around twenty minutes. I felt he was "controlling" me because his voice seemed to emanate from inside my head. He assured me he wasn't.

- Sitting on my bed, I looked across my room and felt on the verge of materializing my ex-girlfriend Gwen by imagining her. I saw a nebula-like, person-size, glitchy distortion in the air and felt startled and looked away from where she would've appeared.

AFTER THE TRIP

Around 5:40 A.M., almost five hours after eating mushrooms—
feeling back and alert and a little frenetic because I wanted to
hurry while I still felt motivated and exhilarated to "leave society," as I'd begun to think was the main message of my trip—I
deleted my Tumblr, my publishing company Muumuu House's
Tumblr, and Muumuu House's Facebook. I considered tweeting
my Gmail password, then tweeted my Facebook password, then
deleted my Twitter and Facebook, feeling both surprised and not.
I'd often "wanted" to but had never actually deleted my accounts
on those websites before.

At 6:01 A.M., my room was lit by doubly indirect sunlight from
that day's 5:58 A.M. sunrise. I deleted my blog and main website,
taolin.info, which I'd posted on almost exclusively in lowercase
letters since 2005, when the URL was reader-of-depressing
-books.blogspot.com, and replaced it with four paragraphs in
capital letters saying I was canceling my UK/Australian obligations and looked forward to being with my family and a few
friends. My message implied I wouldn't be communicating with
anyone else anymore. In paragraph two, I said I was confused,
yawning, and periodically laughing. In paragraph four, I reiterated I was confused and deemed my note "OFFICIAL." The first
paragraph was the longest:

> I DELETED THE 'FRONT PAGE' OF MY GMAIL ACCOUNT . . . ALL THE
> EMAILS. I OFFICIALLY HAVE NO MEMORY. DON'T THINK I HAVE
> ONE OF OYU. I'M SORRY!! LOL. I LOVE MY FAMILY, WILL BE LOOK-
> ING FWD TO SPENDING TIME WITH THEM. AND A FEW FRIENDS.
> EVERYONE ELSE: LOL JESUS GOOD BYE . . . NOT IN A BAD WAY . . .
> OKAY. JESUS . . .

I considered deleting my Gmail account. Increasingly, I felt I needed to rush to fulfill my plan or else it wouldn't happen; as my determination and vision left, I'd probably simultaneously rationalize, I knew, that it was better not to do this; so, using large scissors, I cut the cords connecting the internet to my modem, the modem to my router, my computer to its charger, and other things to other things, feeling only a little self-conscious. I put the cut cords, modem, router, and computer into a black garbage bag, which I put into a public, bus-length garbage container on the street by a construction site two blocks away.

REST OF THE DAY

I slept for around three hours, then walked thirty blocks south to the Apple Store in SoHo to buy another computer. My brother, months earlier, had said he would buy me one for my birthday. I had turned thirty on July 2, one month and three days earlier. After selling me a MacBook Air, an Apple employee said he'd email me the receipt.

Outside, I considered email. Nearly all my communication— with family, friends, acquaintances, media, career-related enti- ties, readers, and combinations of those—occurred by email. When I'd desired deleting my Gmail, I hadn't hurried enough, and the feeling had left. I wanted to want to leave society as much as before; instead, I seemed almost totally pulled back in already. I had bought a computer in a process that began more than a month earlier. I had, from my phone, emailed my editor and agent apologizing—somewhat needlessly, as both had read my all-caps message and emailed their support—and saying I was okay and not canceling my UK/Australian obligations. In the UK, in three days, I would promote and discuss *Taipei*; journalists would talk to me about drugs and young people. I would be deep in society for at least another month, during which I'd become very far from the feeling.

Walking to New York University's library—Bobst Library—to use their computers, I continued thinking about my expending momentum, which had felt unstoppable around twelve hours earlier. Now it seemed so inconvenient to delete my email account that it felt flatly, obviously impossible. Soon, within hours or days, I would forget how it had felt to excitedly believe I'd be living alone in a rural area within weeks or months.

I felt dramatic in a way that itself felt dramatic and false. Why did I feel vaguely ashamed and melodramatic for actualizing change? For trying to leave a life I increasingly disliked, dreaded, and hated? Disposing of my computer—even if on some level I'd known I would get another—and deleting parts of my internet presence were precious, rare behaviors that I didn't want to diminish, belittle, or ignore. I wanted to remember them and how I felt to do them. It was twilight and cloudless—I was in a quiet part of the city, south of the library—and I wanted to stop moving, to kneel and weep, but I kept walking.

NEXT FEW DAYS

As my urge to immediately leave society dissipated, I doubted the wisdom of my plan. It seemed wiser—more effective and earnest and considerate, less frantic and belligerent and crazed—to leave slowly, patiently, and carefully. I began to view my desire not as weakening but transforming—from an isolated outburst to a nuanced, lifelong theme. I didn't want to leave the interconnecting technology of the internet anymore, just parts of it. I regained my Twitter and Facebook accounts, which were impossible, I learned, to delete without thirty days' notice—or, in other words, took thirty days to delete—and reinstated taolin.info in minimal form, without the stream-of-consciousness, retirement note–like message.

I would leave society—its drugs and language and ideas and habits and opinions and websites—incrementally, as a gradual and evolving process. I would use psychedelics, books, my history, my mind, and my body to continue learning and to fill my unconscious with more of my experiences and the mystery and less of culture and its hierarchies, so that I wouldn't sink, like in quicksand but without a directionalized struggle, back into the life I'd once wanted—and had felt, surprisingly and gratefully, empowered—to leave.

②

I don't view my experience as a "bad trip," as I imagine some may think. I view it as my favorite trip that I've had on psilocybin—the one I've given the most attention in my mind and now in print. For me, a bad trip would be one where I hurt myself or others, was imprisoned, or, say, watched TV and ate candy for three hours. I view the trips I share in this book as lessons that were discomforting, portentous, frighteningly intense, and safe. Psychedelic experiences uniquely combine safety and intensity, I've noticed. Other extreme activities—wingsuiting, mixed martial arts—don't seem as low-risk, accessible, feasible, or transcendent.

Without psilocybin, I don't see the imagination brightly with details while awake. I don't realize I'm alien-occupying Tao Lin, sob profusely, delete my websites, feel outside time, announce life changes in typo-dominated blocks of text at 6:01 A.M. or any other time, or discard my computer. Psilocybin removed me from the creodes of my habits and provoked me into long-term change. I'm grateful for all these effects, which aren't all its effects.

McKenna said all psychedelics were similar at low and moderate doses, causing boundary dissolution, increased access to unconscious thoughts and behaviors, compromised ability to repress and ignore memories and problems, and faster and broader and less linear cognition. The effects became idiosyncratic only at high doses. Beyond my experience of 2.5 dried grams is a weirder, less biographical experience, which McKenna said occurred reliably, for a 160-pound person, on 5 dried grams of *Stropharia cubensis*, which was reclassified in 1951 as *Psilocybe cubensis*, or other amounts of other psilocybin-containing species, experienced alone in silence and darkness, or, in the headline form McKenna often said, "5 dried grams in silent darkness."

McKenna stressed that people who hadn't done this, which he called a heroic dose, hadn't experienced psilocybin's full spectrum of effects. I'm unsure if I've eaten a heroic dose, which for me at 125 pounds would be 3.9 dried grams, but I know I haven't in silent darkness (in 2011, 2012, and some of 2013, I often feared being alone in dark places, making it uneasy for me to spend even five minutes in darkness) and that I haven't, except maybe in inchoate ways, experienced the two effects McKenna said occurred on heroic doses.

VISIBLE LANGUAGE

McKenna said heroic doses could impart the ability to produce language into a shared space where it was viewable in 360 degrees by others on psilocybin or DMT. "The thought that is heard becomes more and more intense until, finally, its intensity is such that, with no transition, one is now beholding it in three-dimensional, visual space," he said in "New Maps of Hyperspace" (1984). "One commands it. This is very typical of psilocybin."

He theorized humans could evolve this arguably telepathic behavior; telepathy, in his view, wasn't hearing what others think but seeing what others mean. A species gaining a vaguely magical skill like this seems unlikely and science-fiction-like, which, as I increasingly expect the unexpected, makes it seem like a reasonable prediction. The strange possibility of it reminds me of the J. B. S. Haldane sentence from *Possible Worlds and Other Papers* (1927) that McKenna often paraphrased: "Now, my own suspicion is that the universe is not only queerer than we suppose, but queerer than we *can* suppose." In "The World Could Be Anything" (1990), McKenna theorized humans were a one- or two-gene mutation away from being able, through endogenous DMT, to speak visually. He found an approximate precedent of visible language in nature in octopi, who folded their soft, chromatophored, texture-changing bodies into selective concealment, employing "blushes, dots, stripes, traveling fields" in their "dance of light." McKenna compared human speech—in which one made noises to another, who checked their private dictionary for the meaning of those noises, then made noises back—with octopi communication, in which there is no dictionary:

Both parties are seeing the same thing because my body is my meaning. I become my meaning. And you behold the meaning I have become. I am like a naked thought. Not even a naked nervous system. More naked than that. I am like a naked thought, in aqueous space, unfolding in time. I maintain this is why octopi eject clouds of ink; it's so they can have private thoughts.

The other effect of high-dose psilocybin McKenna described also involved language but was unrelated to visible language. It was the invocation, allowing, or triggering of "a voice in the head," which McKenna called the teaching voice, the Logos, and, most often, "the mushroom." McKenna didn't necessarily believe what the mushroom told him; rather, they dialogued.

THE MUSHROOM

From 1971 until he died, McKenna industriously promoted human re-symbiosis with the mushroom. He ingested it at a range of doses, learned and taught others how to grow it, connected it to human evolution, and mythologized it, outlining and sharing a billion years of its possible history to "the human beings," as he said the mushroom called us. In possibly gracious return, the mushroom shared aphorisms and one-liners and ideas— most notably the theory that all times are harmonic-resonantly related because a fractal wave conditions events on all levels, from milliseconds to centuries—with McKenna, who downloaded selections of these into the public domain as print and spoken-word memes. "Nature loves courage," he quoted the mushroom. "If you don't have a plan, you become part of someone else's plan," he quoted. "Within the mushroom trance, I was informed that once a culture has complete understanding of its genetic information, it reengineers itself for survival," he said in 1982.

Much of what the mushroom told McKenna was answers to his questions. When McKenna asked what it was doing on Earth, it said, "Listen, if you're a mushroom, you live cheap; besides, I'm telling you, this was a very nice neighborhood until the monkeys got out of control." Asked about "the social chaos at the end of history," the mushroom said, "No worry, bro. This is what it's like when a species departs for hyperspace." Asked how to save the world, the mushroom said, "Each person should parent only once." McKenna called this "an astonishing idea." He elaborated in "In the Valley of Novelty":

> This is not zero population growth, this is population falling by 50 percent every twenty years from here on out. If people in the high-tech, industrial democracies would limit themselves to one child, almost immediately the destruction of the Earth's ecosystems and resources would halt. We preach population control in the third world, but the statistics show that to a woman in the first world who has a child, that child will consume between eight hundred and a thousand times more resources in the course of its lifetime than a child born in Bangladesh.

But the mushroom—who was sometimes like Dorothy of Oz, sometimes like a pawnbroker—did not answer all of McKenna's questions. McKenna's approach to it, he said in "New Maps of Hyperspace," was Hasidic. "I rave at it; it raves at me. We argue about what it is going to cough up and what it isn't." In "In the Valley of Novelty," McKenna said the mushroom composed its message "out of bits and pieces of what you already possess" and so "the more you put into your head, the more far-out your trips can be." In "The Psychedelic Option" (1990), he said that, once, during a tumultuous time in his life, he ate mushrooms to try to resolve his personal difficulties. Before the trip, he prepared a question—"Am I doing the right thing?"—and during the trip he asked it. "What kind of a chickenshit question is that?" answered the mushroom. "To ask an extraterrestrial entelechy?" Other things the mushroom would not tell included what happened to human consciousness after death and, as McKenna discussed in a talk in Maui in 1994, what it was for itself:

> The scariest thing to say to it is "Show me what you really are for yourself." At that point, it just begins to come apart, and you can't stand it. After forty seconds of that, you say, "I'm sorry I even asked." You know, reassure me, because you have a sense, my god, this thing *is* what it seems to be. It's a galactic intelligence. It's a billion years old. It's touched ten million worlds. It knows the history of 150,000 civilizations.

EXTRATERRESTRIAL

The idea that *Stropharia cubensis*—and the other two-hundred-plus known species of psilocybin-containing mushrooms—did not originate on Earth was proposed early in McKenna's career, in 1976, and he continued to suggest and promote it throughout his life. The idea came from the mushroom itself, according to McKenna, who quoted it verbatim—"straight transcription," he said in 1983—in the foreword to *Psilocybin*:

> I am old, older than thought in your species, which is itself fifty times older than your history. Though I have been on earth for ages I am from the stars. My home is no one planet, for many worlds scattered through the shining disc of the galaxy have conditions which allow my spores an opportunity for life.

In the two-page quote, the mushroom explained that its nearly immortal body ("only the sudden toxification of a planet or the explosion of its parent star can wipe me out") was a network in the soil with potentially more connections than in a human brain and that it sought symbiosis—a relation of mutual dependence and benefits—with humankind. In its memory was "the knowledge of hyperlight drive ships and how to build them." It would trade this knowledge for a ticket—via humans—to worlds around stars younger and more stable than the sun.

McKenna said one reason he liked to "make this argument about the mushroom and the extraterrestrial" was to show people "how one can see things differently." In the mushroom-focused, penultimate chapter of *True Hallucinations*, he wrote that species with star-travel would "look as they *wished* to look" and that the mushroom, living on dead organic matter, seemed "designed with Buddhist values of noninterference and low environmental impact in mind."

Other evidence, besides the mushroom's own claims, supporting the extraterrestrial-mushroom theory can be found, in McKenna's view, by examining the psilocybin compound. McKenna stressed psilocybin's status as the only known 4-phosphorylated indole in nature. This was unusual, he said in his *tripzine* interview, because "the way biology works is if you have a molecule useful in a biological system, then in other biological systems you will get the same molecule or tiny variants." He called psilocybin "as artificial as a Coke bottle."

◎

McKenna often pointed out that psilocin and DMT are closely related to serotonin, the 25-atom compound that mediates tens of functions in animals. When I contemplate how these three

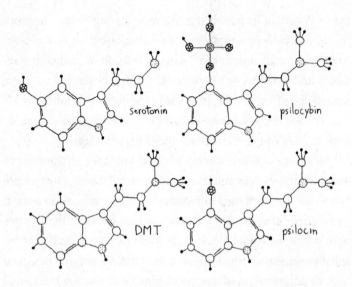

similar compounds, all made from tryptophan, cause three dras-
tically different experiences, I sense this indicates something
about how little of the world a human can detect.

On Earth, serotonin was probably first synthesized three to
four billion years ago by cyanobacteria and later by multicel-
lular plants and fungi before by animals, in which, after neurons evolved around 600 million years ago, it functioned as a
neurotransmitter. It's unknown how old psilocin and its "storage form" psilocybin are, but they've been found only in fungi,
a Kingdom of life that evolved probably at least 2.4 billion years
ago. DMT, which is psilocin minus an oxygen atom, probably
existed more than three billion years ago in small amounts and
then in large amounts around 700 million years ago, when land
plants evolved. Today, DMT is widespread in plants and animals.
In humans, it has been shown or theorized to mediate attention,
orgasm, inflammation, tissue regeneration, immune regulation
of carcinogenesis, neuroprotection in times of low oxygen, spon-

taneous psychedelic states, the perception of dark matter or parallel dimensions, dreams, sleep, childbirth, and death. McKenna was most interested in the experience of smoked DMT, about which, in 1994, he said, "I'm here to tell you that it is real—there *is* a doorway into another dimension."

"Magic" is a seventh word that McKenna and psychedelics helped me define. Before, I associated "magic" with its fantastical meaning of a skill used to harm and heal, its figurative meaning in which auspicious, uncommon events were called magical, and its literal meaning as a synonym for impossible. I avoided using the word because it referred to something I couldn't remember ever experiencing or detecting, though I suspect I did once, as a baby or toddler, before I knew the word, view the world as figuratively and literally magical. Now I associated the word excitedly, earnestly, and specifically with psychedelics—cannabis, which made normal experience magical; psilocybin, which caused behaviors and feelings that seemed previously, personally impossible; and especially DMT, which produced experiences seeming both impossible and unimaginable.

DMT

On October 3, 2015, a Saturday, my internet friend Tracy emailed me in the afternoon saying she'd completed her third extraction of DMT—from chacruna leaves purchased in an herbal market in Iquitos—and would be in New York City from Tuesday to Sunday for the ninth annual Horizons: Perspectives on Psychedelics conference. Would I like to try some of her DMT?

By then I'd smoked DMT three times. The first time was in December 2012, three months after learning of Terence McKenna. A chemistry student (and fan of my writing) had mailed me five self-synthesized doses for $25 in mid-October, and the waxy, orange substance had remained unused in my drawer with my drug stash. I'd avoided it due to feeling that, at this time in my life, while failing more than ever to wean myself off drugs and at times borderline suicidal, my DMT experience would likely be horrifying.

The day the DMT arrived, I'd written "i have dmt on me but want to wait until i feel better via tapering off xanax before using it" in an email to Gwen, my then girlfriend. Ten days later, on

October 29, 2012, Hurricane Sandy caused multiday electrical blackouts in areas of the bottom third of Manhattan, including my apartment building, where Gwen and I and some friends, aware the world was supposed to end soon, had gathered. The coming apocalypse—predicted, it seemed, by the Mayan calendar and, in a way I was only vaguely aware of then, McKenna—plus the hurricane encouraged us to indulge in a nearly weeklong drug binge. (Later, I learned that McKenna argued that humans were, at most, centuries from the end of time but stressed it was not possible to know the end date. He chose a date—December 21, 2012—only so he and others could graph and better contemplate his Timewave theory, it seemed to me. But various people and media had irresistibly latched on to the date, sensationally promoting it as when McKenna believed the world would end.) On November 18, still alive after the eschatologically, meteorologically backed binge, Gwen and I returned, in emails, to the topic of DMT. We wanted to try it but, like the previous month except more, didn't think our timing was wise. I wanted first to "recover more," I said in an email. We decided, as our activity for the night, for one of us to snort heroin and the other to ingest Suboxone—a decision based on what drugs we had—and draw or do something else productive, and so my "recovery" continued. By late December I was "recovering" more than ever.

But I felt bored and uncomfortable one night and was alone and wanted to alter my sensation of existence and had no other drugs. Being inexperienced with smoking (I'd smoked around twenty times ever), I suspected I wouldn't inhale enough DMT to leave the world, and I didn't. Sitting on my bed, I felt disconnected, unpredictably spaced, buzzing sensations that seemed both physiological and psychological. I wasn't sure if the effect was all due to the DMT or also because, in a vigilant state of motionless self-awareness, I was detecting or exacerbating a preexisting condition—some form of amphetamine-related brain damage, internal micro-twitching, or tinnitus-like inner-ear problem. I felt electrified around eight times, at first dreading it, then somewhat desiring it because it obviated, if crudely, my mundane despair and seemed to hint at more of itself. I left my bed once or twice to put more DMT in my glass pipe, which Gwen and I had used three months earlier to smoke a vial of crack that a friend had mailed me. I continued to ineptly and, fearing the full experience, probably self-sabotagingly, with my bad smoking skills, smoke little amounts of DMT, squandering two or three doses.

Seven months later, in July 2013, I tried DMT again. I was less hopeless and using considerably fewer drugs than in December, but still years or many months, I felt, from a mental and physical state recommendable—by myself and, I imagined, most people—for smoking DMT. Seated on my bed with legs dangling off, I kind of impulsively smoked one dose of DMT ("~105mg," according to the chemistry student), inhaling more than in December because, due to increasing cannabis usage, I'd gotten better at smoking. I included a non-psychoactive, half-dried herb with the DMT and I think I inhaled more than once. I tried to remember how much time was supposed to pass—how many seconds or, an especially aloof part of me thought, minutes—until the effects began. I felt I knew this information. Distractedly, I considered how my half-conscious approach to DMT might be accidentally wise or even ideal, since I felt relatively calm. "It goes to my blood, which goes to my brain, so shouldn't it have worked already?" I thought. "Or at least by now?" I wondered what I should be thinking about.

Then something happened that scrambled time and erased my memory, interrupting my continuous experience, since birth, of life, even though I remained conscious. I was suddenly so distant from my prior situation inside a body that I could only sense my life—and the world it was embedded in—as a vague myth, shockingly. The blipped passage of my life—a dot of thirty years in a landscape of billions—seemed like a microscopic span of capillary inside the furred ear of an animal on a planet I was rocketing away from in a vessel that had entered a wormhole and departed the universe.

I arrived, with amazement, in a silvery-gray, bulgingly dimensional, complicatedly pulsating, profoundly unfamiliar-feeling, nonphysical place that seemed ancient, public, and, because I couldn't change perspective, strangely screen-like. It seemed like a dungeon room from *The Legend of Zelda* (1986) experienced from inside the game; things seemed able to enter from left or right, but nothing did. I felt 50,000 years away from where I was before—not in the past or future but in one of the other directions away from the planet of time. At one point I realized with panic that I needed to experience 50,000 years to return to my prior existence, which I couldn't remember; I don't remember how that resolved. Then I was in a sky-like whiteness, densely and glaringly bright. There was something there, and as I tried to comprehend it, it flew away. To chase it, I applied mental pressure behind my eyes. I was trying to use language on it, which I sensed would kill it, which I felt wouldn't happen because of how swift and elusive it seemed in its own environment, outside language.

Parachuting, then, through the night sky of the one planet, out of trillions, that I'd left and forgotten—falling slowly through blank space—around six minutes after smoking, my trip now ending, I sensed I could currently do, and so feel, anything imaginable, as in a lucid dream, which I'd never experienced. I wondered how to take advantage of this opportunity. I didn't want to merely feel "good," didn't want to indulge in sensations from the familiar spectrums of physical pleasure, abstract euphoria, or mindless, pointless joy. What satisfied me unconflictedly? I couldn't think of anything. I didn't want to imagine myself in any situations. I tried to communicate telepathically with a friend, and it seemed to almost work. Finally, as if giving up due to time constraints, I considered sex—deriving sexual pleasure by fantasizing about a situation with an imaginary woman or focusing imagelessly on the sensation of orgasm. I was next aware of myself with my pants half off. I went to my computer and began typing.

A flock of things I'd told myself to remember flew mutely out of view in the sky outside the stuffy cabin of my mind as I focused on one aspect of the experience, trying to type coherently about it:

i should have expected this unexpectedness but by its quality it's definitively not able to be expected

the experience of dmt is unexpected . . . but it's not that . . . it eludes even that definition because naming it would give one the illusion of it having a connection to the word, which would mean allowing oneself to expect it

it's outside language, except by being outside language it can't be described, or to describe it would be to kill it

it's an entity that resists description in language

meaning it's an entity that is the opposite of the bias created by language

it's anti-language

I typed some lines trying to express the inadequacy of what I'd typed—the six lines here that seemed frustratingly and faintly comically irrelevant to what I sensed I most wanted, but still hadn't begun, to remember. Urgently thinking I shouldn't dwell on one topic—especially one in which, having begun analyzing my note-taking, I was already twice removed from the experience—I tried to desultorily address an array of what I was continuously forgetting, like a dream but quicker, dreams being memorable in part because they have familiar things and people. I typed "am i actually the question that someone else is asking to someone else?" in reference to sensing, at one point, that my life was an interrogative communication going from source to recipient. I typed that on DMT it felt possible to leave Earth irreversibly—something I'd told myself was crucial to remember. I typed that maybe I was spreading DNA dimensionally. I couldn't, at my motivation and energy levels, which were low, remember anything else. Over days, I remembered more, but my new memories seemed like language and imagery thrown back at my original memories of the language-proof, higher-dimensional object of what had happened, further obscuring and distorting it.

If death by comet was unexpected, and departing Earth nonphysically like I did on psilocybin was, after decades in the same metaphysical place, beyond unexpected, my experience of smoked DMT was beyond beyond unexpected. It was around two ontological corners. It was closing closed eyes twice, or waking, incredibly, thrice. It was a mental sneeze that kept intensifying, ludicrously, instead of ending in a second. These are ideas I can contemplate to slightly remember how it felt. DMT became extra frightening and notable to me after this trip. It seemed possible I *did* experience 50,000 years, hour by hour, before returning with amnesia of my exile, to my life in the universe, where only five minutes had elapsed.

The next day I uncharacteristically and half-consciously walked forty to fifty blocks without a destination, framing where I lived in two rectangles, and for three or four more days I remained more active, less neurotic, and saner, I felt, than normal. I abstained from pills with unusual ease, spent less time mindlessly refreshing websites, and dwelled less on irrationally conceived problems. I theorized this was because I was deficient in DMT. Three years later, I would find support for this theory while researching glyphosate—Earth's most used pesticide— which made plants, fungi, and microorganisms unable to make three amino acids, including tryptophan, which plants and animals used to make DMT and other compounds.

Eight days after the second time, I smoked DMT a third time. Alone in my room, using the rest of my orange DMT, I smoked less, it seemed, than on July 24, when I had my "50,000 years" experience. Early in the trip, I became distracted by my eyes. I wasn't sure if I wanted to open or close them; trying both, I couldn't discern a difference. After realizing I was wasting time on the visual aspect of my experience, I rushed to focus elsewhere and then at some point experienced "alien sex," as I later, back in the universe, termed it.

On my computer, I typed "all non-experience activity seems pointless, seems worthless, like typing, like recording any info outside oneself" and four more lines before fully realizing I was, again, failing in my note-taking. I refocused and began typing about sex—a topic I'd stressed to myself to remember. I'd sensed the presence of a faceless, bodiless, genderless abstraction, and the experience had felt intensely sexual. This time I did not, like the previous time, feel duly disappointed in myself for thinking about sex while in the imagination; the interaction this time did not seem pleasure-based. I was only terming it "sex" because it had been as intense and relational as sex. Like how I hadn't died during my psilocybin trips when I've felt dead, this wasn't sex. I didn't know what else to type. I'd forgotten most of the trip. I typed that I wanted to smoke more DMT—"as much as it takes, to be in the space it puts me into to completely go there"—but I had none left and didn't try to get more.

Unable, after four or five days, to recall what it felt like, I rarely thought about DMT. I increasingly associated it with my "50,000 years" sensation, which made it seem scary and risky. What if I smoked it and had to wait 50,000 years *again* to return to my life? Hadn't I warned myself that I could go elsewhere permanently? I wanted to recover more before trying DMT again. It was August 2013, the month of my psilocybin trip in the previous chapter.

Twenty-six months later, when Tracy emailed me, I was assuredly recovering from drugs. In the past year, I'd used benzos only around ten times and hadn't used any amphetamines or opiates. Eating healthier, sleeping better, and exercising more, I was less depressed and anxious and more stable and in control of my thoughts and behavior than maybe ever before. I had no excuses not to smoke DMT. I thanked Tracy and said yes to her DMT, which I'd learned a lot about since last smoking it.

$$\oplus$$

N,N-dimethyltryptamine, the simplest psychedelic and commonest in nature, a 30-atom compound made by marine animals, amphibians, reptiles, mammals, and plants, was synthesized in 1931 and found to be psychoactive in 1956 when Stephen Szára injected himself with it in his lab in Budapest, Hungary. In South

America, aboriginals have used it for millennia, insufflating it in snuff preparations and drinking it in ayahuasca, a drink made by boiling or soaking the woody vines of *Banisteriopsis caapi*—or other species from the *Banisteriopsis* genus—with zero or more DMT-containing, or other, plants. Compounds in *Banisteriopsis caapi* inhibit the enzyme that breaks down DMT in the gut before it can reach the brain. "How, one wonders," wrote ethnobotanist Richard Evans Schultes (1915–2001) in 1988, "did these Indians find from the 80,000 species around them these two additives with such extraordinary effects?"

In 1963, City Lights published *The Yage Letters*, a sixty-eight-page "epistolary novel" in the form of twelve letters from William Burroughs (1914–1997) to Allen Ginsberg (1926–1997), a reply, a reply to the reply, and an epilogue. Burroughs, in his letters, described going alone to the Amazon to find yagé—another name for ayahuasca, which is used by people across hundreds of languages—in a 1953 journey that "prefigured," wrote Dennis McKenna in 2012, the McKenna brothers' in 1971. "South America does not force people to be deviants," wrote Burroughs, observing that one could be "queer or a drug addict and still maintain position" and that in the States "*all* intellectuals are deviants." He described two yagé experiences in detail—one seeming painful and unencouraging, one entrancingly hyperdimensional. In the first, Burroughs vomited repeatedly, convulsed with nausea on all fours, twitched uncontrollably, swallowed five Nembutal, had "a chill like malaria," and slept. In the other, which was added to the book in its second edition in 1975, he visited Composite City, a place of "addicts of drugs not yet synthesized" and "blind paranoid chess players," where boys sat in trees "languidly masturbating" and "the unknown past and the emergent future" met in a "vibrating soundless hum." In the morning, still high, this occurred to him: "Yage is space time travel."

DMT became illegal in late 1966, and Terence McKenna first smoked it in early 1967 as an undergraduate at Berkeley. Compared to LSD, it was "so much more alien, raising all kinds of issues about what is reality, what is language, what is the self, what is three-dimensional space and time," he said in an interview in 1988. In "Rap Dancing into the Third Millennium" (1994), he wondered why DMT wasn't "four-inch headlines on every newspaper," why theology hadn't enshrined it as "its central exhibit for the presence of the other in the human world." DMT was physically harmless—its brevity meant the body, which made and used it, knew what to do with it—but still dangerous, McKenna stressed, due to the possibility of "death by astonishment."

COMPOSITE OF COMPOSITES

From 1967 to 1994, McKenna smoked DMT around forty times. In "A Weekend with Terence McKenna," a 1992 workshop, he said when he first did DMT, he "couldn't bring anything out of it," but he went back and kept "working at it." In "Time and Mind" (1990), "The Search of the Original Tree of Knowledge" (1992), "Rap Dancing into the Third Millennium," and the aforementioned workshop, he described composites of his trips. From his four spoken composites, I've made a print composite.

0:00. First toke. Colors brighten, edges sharpen, distant things gain clarity—"there is a sense as though all the air in the room has been sucked out."

0:10. Second toke. You close your eyes and "colors begin racing together" to form a mandalic, slowly rotating, usually yellow-orange thing—"the chrysanthemum," which you break through or, using your glass pipe, require another toke.

0:20. Third toke. The chrysanthemum parts. There's the sound of "a plastic bread wrapper" and a feeling of transition, then "it's as though there were a series of tunnels or chambers that you are tumbling down."

0:40. You burst into "this place." In one composite, McKenna said, "And language cannot describe it—accurately. Therefore I will inaccurately describe it. The rest is now lies." His engagement with this aspect of DMT—that the experience can't be downloaded into as low-dimensional a language as English and so one has to create a story, a series of words conveying as much about the teller as the experience, to talk about it—increased my interest in his DMT accounts. The place is indirectly lit and seems underground—"everything is machine-like and polished and throbbing with energy"—and as you enter there's "a cheer" and then you're "swarmed by squeaking, self-transforming elf-machines" who say "Hooray! Welcome!" And, in McKenna's case, "You send so many and you come so rarely!"

0:50. You're thinking, "Jesus H. Fucking Christ, what is this?" DMT doesn't affect "the part that you call you." You're like before, but the world has been replaced. You're saying, "Jesus, a minute ago I was in a room with some people, and they were pushing some weird drug on me, and, and now, what's happened? Is this the drug? Did we do it?"

1:00. The ball-like elves, made of language, run forward. "These things do not require belief to sustain their

existence—you may doubt, you may deny, yet there they are."
Each elf elbows others aside. "Look at this, take this, choose
me," they say. "And then—and you have to understand they
don't have arms, so we're kind of downloading this into a
lower dimension to even describe it, but—what they do is
they offer things to you." This continues for around three
minutes, during which the elves, speaking an advanced form
of visible language, encourage you not to stagnate in astonishment but to pay attention, to do what they're doing.

4:10. Then—"only 5 percent report this"—"everything stops
and they wait, and you feel like a torch, a spark, lit in your
belly, that begins to move up your esophagus." Your mouth
opens and "language-like stuff comes out." The elves "go
mad with joy."

4:40. "The whole thing begins to collapse in on itself." The
beings move away, and "usually their final shot is they actually wave goodbye." There's "a ripple" and you realize "two
continua are being pulled apart." McKenna said, "And often
it's very erotic, although I'm not sure if that's the word. But
it's almost like sex is the *surface* of which this is the volume."

5:00. "You're raving about it."

7:00. "You can't remember it."

McKenna theorized DMT mediated "the spiral descent into
dream" because, among other reasons, when people smoked
it, their closed eyes darted as if "shoved into deep dreaming."
McKenna had dreams in which he was handed a pipe of DMT,

smoked it, and it worked, implying that one could, at least while asleep, convince oneself to make it. He said everyone's DMT experience would differ, except for how dramatic it would be; once, he introduced a Tibetan lama—"a name that you would recognize, although not one of the top five, but a more wizened, older, stranger character"—to DMT and the lama said it was "the lesser lights," that one couldn't go further without "breaking the thread of return." McKenna concluded:

> This *has* to be taken seriously. In other words, the "it's only a hallucination" thing—that horseshit is just passé. I mean, reality is only a hallucination, for crying out loud, haven't you heard? So that takes care of that—it's only a hallucination. What we've got here, folks, is an intelligent entelechy of some sort that is frantic to communicate with human beings *for some reason.*

WHO ARE THEY?

McKenna called them tykes, fairies, self-articulating sentences, translinguistic elves, friendly fractal entities, elf legions of hyperspace, meme traders, art collectors, and syntactical homunculi. From my three trips, I'd only gotten as detailed as "faceless, bodiless, genderless abstraction" in describing any entities I'd encountered. From his tens of trips, McKenna formed four theories on who they were, which he presented "without judgment" because he was "not sure."

1. Aliens. McKenna said he could imagine aliens that wanted to interact with humans but had ethics prevent-

ing them from landing on Earth, thinking, "Let's analyze these people. Okay—they're kind of hardheaded rationalists, except they have this phenomenon called 'getting loaded,' and when they get loaded, they accept whatever happens to them, so *let's hide inside the load* and we'll talk to them from there, and they'll never realize that we're of a different status than pink elephants."

2. Entities in a parallel continuum. "Call it fairyland, call it the Western Realm, whatever you like, but you don't go there in starships." McKenna called this possibility "friendlier to Pagan notions" and observed that "human folklore in all times and places except Western Europe for the last three hundred years has insisted that these parallel domains of intelligence and organization exist."

3. Dead people. McKenna reached this theory "reluctantly"; due in part to spending his adolescence and early adulthood "getting free from Catholicism and its assumptions," he found it "hair-raising." His evidence for it included that the entities seemed to love us, care for us, and be more aware of us than we of them.

4. Fractal shards of himself, in that if one breaks a mirror, each piece reflects an entire, tiny you. This theory was supported by how McKenna-like the entities were—in their zaniness, contagious glee, and obsession with visual language—but was not supported in other ways, like those examined next.

RICK STRASSMAN

Rick Strassman (b. 1952) studied DMT in an arguably opposite way from McKenna. In 1990, Strassman began the first new, government-funded research in the United States in more than twenty years on the effects of psychedelics on humans. From 1990 to 1995, he administered around four hundred intravenous doses of DMT to sixty volunteers with extensive experience with psychedelics. The results, which he shared and analyzed in *DMT: The Spirit Molecule*, included an unexpectedly high number of encounters with "seemingly autonomous nonmaterial entities" in "freestanding, independent levels of existence." The entities were called Jokers, clowns, "the entities or whatever they are," cartoonlike people, aliens, guides, helpers, reptiles, mantises, bees, spiders, cacti, stick figures, and, by at least one person, elves. When people opened their eyes, the hospital room overlapped with the DMT reality.

In *DMT*, which was published in December 2000, eight months after McKenna died, Strassman wrote that, due to Burroughs's frightening accounts of its effects, the compound had remained "relatively obscure" until the mid-1980s, when McKenna began "praising it publicly and lavishly." Strassman was familiar with McKenna—in a footnote he said he'd visited Terence in Hawaii and that Terence had estimated 5 percent of people he'd given DMT showed "nearly no effect," a number matching Strassman's study in which three of the sixty volunteers were unaffected—but most of the volunteers, who had little contact with one another, were not. Strassman often asked volunteers if they were familiar with "popular accounts of DMT-mediated encounters with elves or insectoid aliens"; few, "if any," were; therefore, he argued, the entities did not seem to be "a type of mass hysteria or a self-fulfilling prophecy."

In a 2013 essay titled "DMT Research from 1956 to the Edge of Time," Andrew Gallimore and David Luke wrote that around half in Strassman's study had reported "travelling to normally invisible worlds and meeting an array of peculiar beings." The essay argued that this might not be "a later counter-cultural affectation" but "a core feature" of the phenomenology of DMT because it had also featured in the first DMT tests on humans, in 1958 and 1959, before cultural input on DMT existed. In 1958, in Budapest, Stephen Szára injected thirty volunteers, mostly doctors from the National Institute for Mental and Nervous Diseases, where he worked, with 0.7 mg/kg, or around 50 milligrams, of DMT. Of the surviving accounts, one person said the room became "full of spirits," one saw "two quiet, sunlit Gods," and one encountered "strange creatures, dwarfs or something." In a study done a year later, a "33-year old psychotic" given 50 milligrams of DMT intramuscularly met "horrible" "orange people" who were "not human."

One of the more shocking experiences in Strassman's study was by a volunteer named Ken. It isn't a representative experience, but I share it here as counterpoint—equally appalling but tonally opposite—to McKenna's experiences.

[Ken] settled down at about the 5-minute point, but grimaced and shook his head. Within a couple more minutes he took off his eyeshades and stared straight ahead. His pupils remained large, so Laura and I sat quietly, waiting for him to come down further. At 14 minutes, looking shaken but keeping some composure, he started [talking],

There were two crocodiles. On my chest. Crushing me, raping me anally. I didn't know if I would survive. At first I thought I

*was dreaming, having a nightmare. Then I realized it was really
happening.*

I was glad he didn't have the rectal probe[*] in place, this
being a screening day.

Tears formed in his eyes, but stayed there.

"It sounds awful."

*It was awful. It's the most scared I've ever been in my life. I
wanted to ask to hold your hands, but I was pinned so firmly I
couldn't move, and I couldn't speak. Jesus!*

In *DMT*, Strassman also described his two-year, remarkably
persistence-requiring ("I called every day for the next ten days,
asking for the fax."), Kafkaesque ("The DEA would approve nei-
ther Dave's request to make DMT nor my Schedule I permit to
possess it until the FDA approved the protocol. The FDA couldn't
give me permission until I possessed the drug and tested it for
safety.") process, involving syncopated interactions with an ethics
committee, a scientific advisory board, the FDA, the DEA, and
others, of getting approval to do the studies. Strassman shared
this narrative to show it was possible.

His research, which eventually included psilocybin, ended in
1995 after, among other difficulties, his ex-wife was diagnosed
with cancer, his Buddhist monastic community began criticizing
his research and "withdrawing their personal support," and he
was denied permission to relocate the research setting to somewhere less egregious than a loud hospital, which in an interview
he called "the most distasteful, in some ways, possible place for
people to have huge trips."

* The temperature-measuring probe, which only one person refused, was
around one-eighth of an inch in diameter and, made of rubber-coated wire,
"quite flexible." Strassman wrote that it "went in about four to six inches and
rarely caused any discomfort, except in those with hemorrhoids."

Near the end of his book, Strassman, a medical doctor, wrote that he "had little interest in or knowledge about alien encounters" before the DMT study and that, after, he felt required to include "contact" as a phenomenon mediated by "high levels of brain DMT."

㉔

At around 7:00 P.M. on October 10, 2015, one week after emailing me her DMT offer, Tracy arrived at my apartment after spending her day at the psychedelics conference in a church by Washington Square Park. We'd met online in 2007 through our blogs and since then had communicated tens of times, including in 2009, when a website asked me for recommendations and I chose, with four other things, Tracy's Microsoft Paint blog, calling it "my favorite collection of one-panel 'comics' online or in print," but we'd never met in person. I'd learned of Tracy's interest in psychedelics the previous year, when she noticed my *Vice* column and emailed to say she was "quite possibly the biggest Terence McKenna fan in the world" (which she qualified with "but probably not? idk") and that McKenna was why she was studying altered states of consciousness in college. After graduating, she'd traveled and studied in Peru for three months, returned to the States with dried leaves of chacruna, or *Psychotria viridis*, and done an "acid-base extraction" on them—a method involving lye, naphtha, coffee filters, ammonia, a freezer, and distilled water—to isolate their DMT in a crystal form.

Tracy said I should smell the white DMT, which was in a contact lens case. I said I wanted to focus first on not sneezing. She showed me two tabs of LSD in the case's other side and said she didn't like LSD. She held the case toward me and I accidentally exhaled, causing a little DMT to go in the air. It smelled like mothballs, which I hadn't smelled since childhood, making the scent distinctive and familiar. To smoke it, I'd made a plastic-aluminum device—a two-liter bottle with the bottom replaced with foil—into which vaporized DMT could be stored until I unscrewed the cap and inhaled it all at once.[*] I'd learned how to make this by searching "how to best smoke DMT" on You-Tube and clicking the second result—"How I've Smoked (DMT) Dimethyltryptamine"—which had more than 450,000 views.

We discussed Tracy's new job, writing for a local newspaper, then planned what to do after my trip. I said I wanted to drink iced coffee and type about my experience; in my email response seven days earlier, the previous Saturday, I'd mentioned wanting to "focus on typing about the experience for like hours" right after my trip. Tracy said that, in return for the DMT, she would at least like for me to briefly tell her what happened before she left. I agreed to this plan, which seemed more than fair.

Tracy used my wood-handled pocketknife, which I'd used, mostly to cut food, almost daily for around two years, to transfer DMT to a crater of foil. As we taped the foil to the bottle, part of me somewhat automatically, as a person who routinely considered each situation's worst possibilities, felt paranoid that Tracy was there to poison me. It seemed unwise and unnecessary to not share this intuition, which I felt could lighten the mood. From what I could discern of her sense of humor based on our online interactions and her Microsoft Paint art—one drawing was of an olive-eyed face with the caption "i have olive eyes im scared"; another was a girl with two cats, ice cream, and other things stacked on her head, her arms around a cat and a mon-

---

[*] I don't recommend plastic or aluminum to smoke anything because, I later learned, both will vaporize to some degree. I recommend glass.

key, and the caption "i have it all"—I felt Tracy might enjoy my revelation.

Seeming maybe a little taken aback but not unnerved, Tracy said she wasn't going to kill me. This was really DMT. I said I believed her fully, which I did. I said I wanted to go for a walk first. We decided to smoke cannabis before going outside.

We walked east three blocks, turned 180 degrees, and walked back toward my apartment. We discussed Holotropic breathing, Kundalini yoga, and Weston A. Price (1870–1948), a Canadian dentist who visited fourteen non-modern societies in the 1930s, photographing teeth and studying diets. Price published his findings—that aboriginals prized foods that modern people shunned, like animal organs and animal fats, and that modern food resulted in cumulative degeneration—in *Nutrition and Physical Degeneration* (1939), which included more than 150 photos of Native Americans, aboriginal Australians, Eskimos, and other dietarily non-modern people, like the isolated Swiss of the Lötschental Valley. Physical degeneration was body-wide, but Price focused on facial degeneration. Modern people can't fit all thirty-two teeth in their mouths in a neat, aligned manner not, I learned, due to breeding between races—as some, Price observed, had theorized—but multigenerational malnutrition. Aboriginals, to name one difference, began feeding women nutrient-dense food—egg yolks, liver, seafood—for up to six months before marriage, then during and after pregnancy.

The more time and physical scale, from galaxies to microbes to molecules, I included in my model of the world—and the more I absorbed the work of Price, McKenna, Harrison, and others who viewed deep time and aboriginals and nature with curiosity and enthusiasm, as obvious sources of knowledge—the more complex and, surprisingly, less confusing the world became. In the past, it had seemed impossible to learn accurate information about health and diet; now it increasingly seemed wise to trust aboriginal diets, which had developed and optimized over tens of thousands of generations outside the influence of publicly owned companies, which seemed to be the main influence on what twenty-first-century modern people ate and viewed as healthy. Aboriginal ways with food—the calm result of millions of years of nature-embedded evolution—had not been warped by a century and trillions of dollars' worth of advertising, marketing, branding, and packaging from thousands of corporations.

The effects of society-wide degeneration included pain, confusion, dark humor, and, it seemed to me, a kind of restlessness. The more suffering that was built into the human body, the deeper human consciousness—squirming and uncomfortable inside malformed bodies—burrowed into the imagination, reaching stranger places and downloading subtler and more complex and grotesque and startling ideas and behaviors and art and lives into the universe. Physical degeneration, which in its current thread began with agriculture at least 12,000 years ago and worsened significantly in the twentieth century with non-organic farming, factory farms, processed food, thousands of synthetic compounds, and depleted soil—the terrestrial source of nutrition—seemed to be one factor that encouraged individuals, through discomfort and dissatisfaction, to invent things, start companies, write novels, cause wars, explore unknowns, theorize transcosmically.

In college, I'd been surprised to read a line of backstory in Lorrie Moore's fractal novel *Anagrams*, which was made of four stories that were ideally, said Moore in an interview in 2001, "thought of as little satellites orbiting" the short novel ending the book, revealing that a character had, as a child, "nightly pressed her front teeth hard against the heel of her hand, to push them back: orthodontia for the poor and trailered." I didn't grow up in a trailer and had gotten braces like most of my peers, but I also, like Moore's character, had pushed my teeth—and other parts of my skull—with the heels of my hands at night in bed. After recognizing the behavior in Moore's fiction, I realized many children probably felt intuitively compelled to push their teeth into their mouths, to try to change their skull shape, not just me. After reading *Nutrition and Physical Degeneration* in November 2014, I finally realized why.

My teeth and tongue had always felt too big—especially before having eight teeth pulled so the remaining twenty-four could non-snaggledly fit—for my mouth, which felt small behind lips that seemed often almost numb with oversizeness. I'd assumed my face felt bad because I wasn't as healthy as other children, or that this was just how life felt—mocking, cramped, obnoxious, achingly awkward. I'd assumed it was normal for most people to have buckteeth, crooked bites, crowded mouths, and other facial problems. Now I was glad and empowered to learn it wasn't normal. It was because our upper and lower jaws, among other body parts, were thwarted expressions of human DNA—were degenerate—and had been, in this diet-induced way that could be reversed in future generations, for only, depending on the person, 1 to, at most, around 480 generations, "only" because the human species was at least 11,200 generations old.

Back in my room post-walk, I said I was going to type about how I felt, as per my DMT checklist, which I'd created the day before, stipulating that, before smoking DMT, I would (1) type about how

I feel, (2) meditate, (3) breathe. "Typing how I feel now," I typed on my MacBook Air, which I'd purchased twenty-six months earlier. The past week, I'd sometimes anticipated my upcoming DMT trip causing me to do what would seem, from my current perspective, deeply inconvenient—isolating myself in some permanent way, deleting my email and other accounts, disposing of my computer, phone, keys, and/or cards—but which, post-DMT, would seem irresistible. "I feel kind of disoriented and blank," I typed in notes.rtf, a file I'd typed in 97 to 99 percent of days since October 28, 2013. "Earlier I thought it would be funny and interesting if I felt blank during this and maybe that is making me feel a little blank."

I told Tracy I was going to sit and breathe. I entered my DMT tunnel, which I'd also created the day before. In the afternoon, using my black-sheeted mattress as a movable wall, I'd created a DMT corner, which, at night, I'd tightened and decreased into a tunnel, where I'd slept on my yoga mat with my childhood blanket; supine in darkness, around midnight I'd considered how I'd had a hedonistic trip (on DMT), an alien-sex trip (on DMT), and a "leave society" trip that was briefly messianic (on psilocybin). These seemed to be possibilities I'd gotten through. Now I would try to have an exploratory, information-gathering trip.

After breathing cross-legged, I stood and breathed with swinging arms to further oxygenate and calm myself. I smoked another hit of cannabis, which hadn't been part of the plan. Despite this transgression, I felt in a good, somewhat playful, childlike, non-despairing, mostly unworried, ready mood. I reviewed my post-DMT plan:

1. Tell Tracy what I saw

2. Type account

3. Drink caffeine while typing if desired

4. Try going into third-person if desired

Tracy brought the plastic bottle into the DMT tunnel, and I felt not ready anymore. I felt a little like hiding and being alone and quitting, though I was smiling and vaguely giddy. Remembering that some volunteers in Strassman's study had floundered and spasmed, I wondered aloud how to position my body. Tracy suggested sitting with legs stretched ahead. I decided on cross-legged. I said I wanted to verbally rehearse what was about to happen—I would heat the foil, the DMT would vaporize, I'd inhale air, exhale air, unscrew cap, inhale DMT, give Tracy the bottle, close eyes—but Tracy said no, I shouldn't overthink it. In my indecision, I felt grateful for the confidently stated instruction, but I wanted to talk more to expend restless energy that was becoming anxiety, so I kept talking and we seemed to argue a little on if a step-by-step run-through was desirable or not. Purposefully stalling, I said things to sustain a mirthful and humorous rapport, within which I would gradually feel calmer. Tracy was sometimes laughing, which calmed me. I felt moderately stoned and was also sometimes laughing.

As I self-consciously heated the foil, I felt unsure what to say or think. We were suddenly quiet. I was about to ask if the flame should touch the foil when Tracy said not to touch the flame to the foil. I realized I could be mute—Tracy would talk and I could zone out socially. The disquietingly serious scent of DMT, startlingly and humblingly mnemonic of other worlds, cast doubt on normal reality—a room in a city in human culture on a planet in space and time.

Unscrewing the cap, I distractedly occupied my mind and supported my behavior with historical precedent indicating a thread of character by remembering times I'd unhesitatingly behaved courageously. In grade school when I spit on a minivan on a dare and was sent to the principal's office. When I was ten or eleven and jumped off a roof and didn't get hurt.

0:00. I inhaled the cloud of DMT with a full, satiating breath in four seconds, then screwed the cap back on. It was around 8:05 P.M. "Now hold it in as long as you can," said Tracy, taking the bottle. Wincing a little from the intensity of my upper-body situation, I nodded mutely with shoulders abnormally high, above extra-filled lungs.

0:08. Closing my eyes, I unconsciously turned five to ten degrees toward my computer, which for the past eight minutes twenty-three seconds had been recording a video, which Tracy and I had agreed was a good idea. Sensing the need to immediately concentrate because many complex things were beginning to happen, I quickly brought my hands up into prayer position, the sides of my index fingers touching my lips, and remained motionless like this—straight-backed, hands clasped. With two exceptions, which I remembered later in the night, I have no memory of the next four minutes fifty-two seconds.

0:17. My motionlessness ended with my head tilting slightly back, away from my hands, which remained in a self-canceling position, lessening my sensation of my body. I looked like I was on a magic carpet flying ahead.

0:22. I exhaled audibly through my nose. My eyes trembled wildly, exhibiting rapid-eye movements behind closed, scrunched lids. My expression was earnest, engaged, brow-furrowed, challenged.

0:34. My hands disengaged prayer position and somewhat distractedly rested palms-down on the yoga mat. I leaned forward, as if landing or arriving somewhere. Tracy left the DMT tunnel.

0:41. I laughed a little. I fully covered my face with both hands, then laughed quietly, almost mischievously, through my hands. After five seconds I removed my hands, revealing a grinning face with open, alert eyes. My hands returned to prayer position and bowed forward and back in front of my amused face as if busily, enjoyably praying.

0:56. "Interesting," I said in response to returning to an intenser, tinier-detailed version of a DMT place I'd visited before and had mostly forgotten until then—a place with squiggly, bulging, self-spiraling, involuting, organismic shapes that I experienced visually, auditorily, and ontologically. I was one of them, it seemed, while here—an internally bending, screw-like, purply gray entity, whorling into and out of myself. I heard strange, bouncy, rubbery noises that felt somehow sexual. My first time here, I'd lingered maybe half a minute. Now I was zooming through in seconds. Worlds blurred past. My left eyebrow—which I later learned I normally don't move without also moving my right eyebrow—briefly went, by itself, higher on my forehead than I've ever seen it.

1:00. "It's more interesting than . . . I anticipated," I said while experiencing the unengageable blur in a visceral, severely preoccupying way. I began deep breathing—something I'd been doing more the past year—and slowly moving my upper body forward and back. Calmly swaying in an unconsciously rhythmic, uninhibited manner with wide-open, receptive, alert eyes, I looked like I was seated in active, satisfying contemplation of fun and poignant topics.

1:29. "The question is do I want to keep breathing—" I said conversationally, sounding like I was talking to myself.

"Yes," said Tracy in a robotic voice.

"—or not," I said, finishing my thought, showing no reaction to Tracy's voice.

"Yes," repeated Tracy.

I suddenly stopped swaying. My demeanor changed from calm to stricken and suspicious. My eyeballs turned toward Tracy's voice on the other side of the mattress. Seeming to forget the voice—and become reengaged with something outside the universe—I began swaying again, a little less uninhibitedly than before.

1:52. "This is something that is . . . interacting," I said slowly. My hands were relaxed in front of me in the air—the left holding the right like a dog's mouth holding a rubber toy—moving up and down as if steadying myself while deep in thought.

"I'm in . . . ter," I said very slowly, squinting one eye in acute contemplation.

"Yes, just go with it," said Tracy.

". . . act," I said, and rested my left hand on a gray-socked foot. My right hand, alone in the air, moved rhythmically up and down, as if conducting my concentration. "Go with it," I said in a tone of agreement and approval. I nodded affirmatively. My eyes glanced Tracyward, and I put my hands together in prayer, then rested them palms-down on the yoga mat. I hung my head down, seeming overwhelmed. "Tracy," I said, and looked suspiciously in her direction.

"Tracy," I said in a voice like I thought I might be alone.

"Uh-huh?"

"Where are you?"

"I'm here."

I looked extremely perplexed for three seconds. "I forgot about you," I said, waving my right arm in her direction while slightly hunchbacked. "Where are you? Where are you?"

"I'm here," said Tracy.

I leaned my upper body toward her. "Can you come here?"

"Mhm," said Tracy, and entered the DMT tunnel.

"Should I touch you?" I mumbled with a bewildered, confused expression while perceiving Tracy with difficulty and awe as a slightly reptilian, huge-eyed entity, radiating spiky light, like an animated, Kirlian photograph. She held my right hand with her left hand.

3:14. I stared in concentration at our hands. In overwhelmed confusion, I briefly closed both eyes, then opened my left then right eye and glared suspiciously up at Tracy, who was kneeling, sitting on her feet. I was still cross-legged. I appeared to be concentrating as much as possible in response to being confronted with an intensely novel somethingness that continually remained astonishing and incomprehensible.

"This feels weird," I said, moving our hands up and down a little, then suddenly took my hand away and stopped looking at Tracy. My eyes became round and calm and I swayed backward, as if dodging something while flying. I briefly stared at my hand in extreme, shocked confusion.

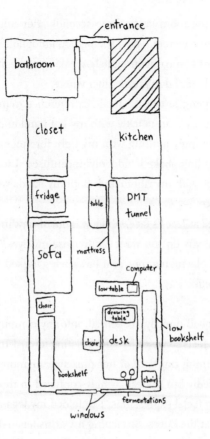

"Close your eyes, close your eyes," said Tracy. "Breathe. Keep your eyes closed." After a delay, I sat straight, closed my eyes, and breathed, as if hypnotized. My upper body swayed forward and back. I opened my eyes, looking baffled. "Do I *want* to close my eyes?" I said in a conversational tone, as if normally talking to Tracy.

"Yes. Close your eyes."

"Why?"

"You'll see," said Tracy.

My eyes remained open, though I hadn't seen or been

aware of my room since three seconds after inhaling. My behavior in concrete reality seemed on autopilot, like it was a small part of me unconsciously speaking while most of me was elsewhere. I don't remember where.

"I'm going to test it," I said in reference to [unknown], scratching my chin quickly with my left hand and pointing left at seemingly nothing with my right forefinger. My face, almost smiling, looked suddenly unconfused. I touched my right cheek with my right hand. Both my hands were touching my face.

I stared at Tracy's face, which was out of view in the video.

"Wait, why do you want me to close my eyes?" I said in an almost playful manner, as if I was being tricked in a harmless, gamelike way.

4:24. I looked directly, it seemed, into my computer's camera. "This feels so weird," I said, scooting toward Tracy a little while seeming unaware of her presence anymore. I looked complicatedly but undespairingly confused in three or four successive facial expressions. I unfolded my legs in front of me, bent at the knees. Stretching my arms leisurely in front of me, my right hand grazed Tracy's knee as she stood and, saying, "Yeah, just close your eyes," left the tunnel. My eyes were widely open. I looked content, spirited, and extra alert. "Breathe," I said confidently to myself, inhaling and exhaling deeply and peacefully.

4:49. "So this is gonna be," I said with an excited expression, swaying forward and back with conscious, thinking, relaxed eyes, then made a small laughing noise. "This . . . should be . . . this experience should be . . . *different*," I said, and suddenly looked bored. "Than my normal," I said, looking engaged and stimulated again.

5:00. I folded my legs in and, using my right hand to gesture while talking, put my left hand on the yoga mat for support and kneeled, saying, "Experience," then stood. "Of day-to-day life . . . drawing," I said while vaguely recognizing an amorphous, context-less thing as my drawing table, where I drew standing because I had hip and back pain that I suspected was due at least partly to sitting too much. "My daily life," I said, looking at the table, which seemed to float blurrily in empty space.

"Do you still feel it? Are you still there?"

"Am I . . . still . . . under . . . the . . . effects . . . of . . . it?"

"Uh-huh," said Tracy.

"Yeah. Yeah. 'Cause this normally . . . this isn't what I experience. I don't think this is what I normally . . . I experience each . . . day. 'Cause each day," I said, and laughed a little. "Twenty-four hours in a day, right?"

"Mhm," said Tracy.

"There's twenty-four . . . *hou*rs in a day. And there's 360 degrees," I said, then walked out of the DMT tunnel and saw smoking paraphernalia on the floor.

6:18. "Yeah, so I smoked a drug!" I said in an excited, relatively loud voice, realizing there was an explanation for whatever had happened—which I couldn't remember—and was still happening.

"Are you . . . back? Are you back?"

"Obviously . . . not . . . yet," I said, enunciating words as if speaking them for the first time. "I'm not back *yet* . . ."

"But kind of?"

". . . 'cause I smoked a drug and, yeah, the effects are wearing off . . . 'cause I'm remembering . . . ," I said to myself, unsure exactly who Tracy was and why she was there, on the sofa. From a formless somethingness, plus time divisions and a spatial aspect, and now this, I began foggily remembering life. I was in a dense city . . .

"You're starting to feel normal again?"

"More normal," I said distractedly while sensing my situation—amid miles of buildings—as intriguingly science fictional. At first, aware only of a blobbily pixelated, strangely patchwork, detaillessly shifting image, I'd thought I was insane, that, shockingly and appallingly, I'd somehow gone insane, but now I was realizing that I was going to be able to sufficiently perceive or re-create reality to not be insane.

Tracy laughed.

"Yeah, 'cause I used to stand here and draw. I used to stand there and draw," I said, then noticed the computer filming.

7:05. "Why is . . . what's this?" I said with audible, almost quivering fear. "Recording?" I said in a scared, confused, ambivalently curious voice.

Tracy laughed loudly. "You don't remember that you recorded it?"

I stared helplessly at the computer.

"Sit down, and chill out," said Tracy.

NEXT THREE MINUTES

"No, I don't remember this part," I said in a shaky voice, pointing at the computer. I was standing, so my head was out of view on the screen.

"Okay," said Tracy in a tone indicating it was fine—not something to panic about—to not remember.

"I don't remember that," I said firmly, then laughed a little. I barely remembered my own life. "I just felt paranoid," I said, and made a frightened, surprised, laugh-like noise.

"When? There?"

"Yeah," I said, less as an answer than to stall so I could think.

"When we were doing the tape?"

"Yeah," I said distractedly. "Earlier did I feel paranoid of you?"

"*To* me, you mean? Did you seem paranoid to me?"

"No," I said, confused. "I suspect—sus-suspected you of doing something to me . . . earlier."

"Oh, you weren't joking? I thought you were kidding. You said, 'Are you going to kill me?' and I said no. I thought you were joking." Tracy laughed a little.

"I . . . *was* . . . joking," I said in a serious voice.

"Okay," said Tracy lightly. "I know."

She coughed. "Sit down," she said.

"I *was* joking," I repeated, unsure what this meant.

"Yeah, I know," said Tracy.

"So you didn't *kill* me," I said with a strange emphasis on "kill," making it sound difficult to pronounce.

"No," confirmed Tracy. "Is that what you wanted?" she said in a voice that sounded, in my DMT-stoned state, which felt as if I'd woken from a long nap into a moderate LSD trip, like I'd unwisely desired something and gotten it.

"I didn't want you to kill me," I said in a quiet voice, half to myself, still somewhat assuming, due to a lack of other possibilities, that I was dead.

"What did you see?" said Tracy. "Did you see something?"

"I'm back now?" I said in a confused voice. "I'm not back yet."

"Okay," said Tracy.

"Well . . . I'm thinking, like, Jesus, that was . . . weird," I said quietly.

Tracy laughed.

"Where's my . . . I need to type it," I said, indicating I wanted to type notes. Had I had some sex-like experience in another dimension with an entity who was now on my sofa?

"Want me to help you?"

"Help me type it," I said, looking for my computer.

"No, like—" said Tracy.

"Write it," I said, looking around for writing materials.

"No, just chill out for like two minutes."

I kneeled then sat on the floor.

"Yeah, sit," said Tracy.

We were out of view in the video.

"You didn't kill me," I said in a voice like I was reconfirming something I was glad seemed true, then laughed a little, sounding less scared for the first time since noticing the computer recording.

"No, you're alive," said Tracy.

"Okay," I said.

"You should yell 'I am alive!' "

"What?" I said absently. "How many minutes . . . since I smoked?"

"I don't know," said Tracy, and appeared in the video facing the computer.

"Let's see if . . ." she said, looking at the screen.

My left eye and half my forehead entered the video and I said, "Seventeen minutes?!" in an incredulous voice as Tracy said the same thing calmly. "But I don't know when you turned it on exactly," she said, then estimated, accurately, that I'd smoked around ten minutes earlier.

I turned my computer toward me and started typing. My face looked calm and energetic. Tracy, behind me, bent at her waist, spied on what I was typing. "Sorry," she said after around six seconds, then laughed a little at herself, stopped looking at the screen, and, adding, "I'm so nosy," moved away, onto the sofa.

I turned my head distractedly and briefly toward her, unaware of her spying or what she'd just said. "Ten minutes? Has it really been . . . ten minutes?" I said with a manic, distracted expression, turning back to the screen, where in notes.rtf I was typing about time—how whatever happened, which I still couldn't remember, hadn't felt at all like ten minutes.

"Wait, were you just watching this?" I said suspiciously, finally processing what she'd said.

"No, I can't see," she said innocently.

I carried my computer into the DMT tunnel.

"Well, you're going to make it public anyway," she said in a playful, singsongy voice. Then she laughed in a manner sounding malicious and threatening. Within seconds, I reinterpreted her tone as openly and confidently antagonistic and sarcastic, which made me feel very paranoid. My face in the video seemed distressed and worried.

NEXT TEN MINUTES

In the DMT tunnel, I tried to type about my experience but mostly just stared at the screen. Tingly sensations across my torso made me sometimes think I'd been stabbed, was bleeding. Sometimes I closed my eyes and tried to remember, or somehow figure out, what happened. Had something been so embarrassing or unseemly or offensive or horrific that I immediately repressed the entire experience? Sometimes I crawled or walked out of the tunnel to briefly, indirectly query Tracy, returning each time to the computer with more, new paranoia-fueling words to mentally replay and use in my distraught model building.

My mind collaged theories desperately and I strongly invested my belief in each and not all were nightmarish. Some were excitingly auspicious and, especially between theories saying I was going to jail for decades, powerfully and humblingly relieving. My internal state went from terror to elation. With each oblique exchange of language, my models of what had happened and was happening changed significantly. Tracy's intonation ranged widely—from mildly inflected to suddenly detached and monotone to entrancingly, theatrically, inventively expressive. In my confused state, her nuanced voice was dense with unspoken meaning and secondary, connotative features, most of which I interpreted self-defeatingly. Unaware I normally wore glasses, I didn't attribute the frustratingly painting-like, splotchy appearance of things to my defective vision; I projected all my suspicions onto Tracy's low-resolution form without knowing I was taking something blurry and imagining the details inaccurately, in overly pessimistic (mostly) or optimistic (sometimes) ways.

I felt I needed to elicit information from Tracy—that could help me remember what happened—without revealing I remembered nothing and was at times petrified with fear. At first, I was able to control my face to make it look relatively stoic and inscrutable, but then I began to feel overheated and tense and self-conscious. I realized my face had begun to look accurately terrified and defeated and vulnerable, that I was flustered and blushing. Sometimes, doubting my innocence, I thought that maybe Tracy hadn't planned this but that I'd unexpectedly done something—while blacked out, maybe—deserving her coldness and disdain, that she was telling the truth and was even being generous by not, for example, calling the police or leaving, but staying to talk. Two or three times, she asked if I was ready to share anything, if there was anything at all I could say, and I responded I was still thinking. "So," I said after around five minutes. "How long after I smoked it did you . . ."

"What?" said Tracy.

". . . try to talk to me?"

"I didn't try to talk to you," she answered after a pause. "You talked to me," she said in a voice that sounded subtly and very accusatory, increasing my paranoia. She seemed to be assuredly manipulating the story to her advantage, to frame me. She said I talked to her "during," which confused and troubled me.

"But I was over here," I said, beginning to reveal and promote my side of the story, aware the video was recording all the audio in the room, to complicate Tracy's story that she was trying, I felt, to make the official one.

"Yeah, well, you called me over," she said. "You called me over," she repeated, as if cementing this improvised reality. She said I'd been speaking very slowly, that I'd said, "This is interesting . . . something is . . . I am interacting with something," which didn't seem incriminating but, in my paranoid state, instead of mollifying my fear, added a dauntingly unsettling, horror-movie-like eeriness.

My sensation of victimization, of being targeted and masterfully defeated, already higher than probably ever before in my life, increased considerably at one point when Tracy, with what sounded like gleeful delight, said, "You're going to see in the video exactly what happened. It's going to be so funny to watch."

In the last three minutes of this ten-minute period, I walked to the refrigerator to get my bottle of iced coffee, which contained 270 milligrams of caffeine. In my fluctuating paranoia, like a pendulum, I felt temporarily okay. Then I noticed Tracy handwriting notes—seeming like a veteran, diligent journalist, seated with straight posture on my sofa—and part of me assumed she was producing incriminating information to use against me. Her notes would be viewed as factual evidence in court and by editors of magazines—something that had always seemed dubious to me, since obviously a journalist would also concoct notes if they were going to lie in print, but I understood this was how things worked, that Tracy's notes could be as damning as video footage, so I felt extra self-conscious of my words. "It just feels like I'm leaving, I'm going from a place of nothing to this," I said, feeling like I was focusing on this aspect of the experience, which I knew I'd already discussed, primarily to suppress or distract from a terrible memory, and that Tracy was scrutinizing me for inconsistencies. Almost trembling in fear, I sensed I was more annoying and repulsive to Tracy than she was showing—that she was professionally restraining her real emotions. "Now it's beginning to feel normal, like everything's normal," I said, standing by my refrigerator, aware I was at least partially lying. I asked Tracy when I'd called her over and she said, "I think after like five minutes."

For some reason this made me feel less paranoid. Then she said, "Actually, I'm trying to write down what I saw, 'cause it was very interesting and unexpected." I heard the last four words as "very interesting from my perspective" and felt dread, curiosity, and, mostly, terror. I returned with coffee to the DMT tunnel and stopped the video at twenty-nine minutes twenty-seven seconds, scared of what it had recorded. I could delete it, I knew. In Photobooth, you pushed Delete to delete forever, it seemed. If the video was incriminating, and I deleted it to save myself, that seemed immoral. But deleting ambiguous information that was going to be distorted into damning evidence seemed like self-defense. During thoughtless-seeming seconds, I deleted the video.

NEXT SEVEN HOURS

After deleting the video at around 8:28 P.M., my paranoia increased further. More than once during the next eighty minutes, which were not recorded, I became aware of my legs trembling from, it seemed, fear and other psychological reasons. To a third person, Tracy and I would have appeared to be having a slow, surreal, sometimes psychotherapeutic, sometimes tense conversation. I was in the tunnel, I think, for most of this unrecorded period, struggling to determine who she was and what had happened. At around 9:48 P.M., I secretly began recording a second video. "What other drugs did you make me smoke?" I asked Tracy, almost directly accusing her of poisoning me. She said it was pure DMT, nothing mixed. We continued talking, and I continued, as I had in various forms since noticing my computer recording the first video, suspecting her of being, among other possibilities:

- A CIA agent. In the past five years, I'd discussed illegal drugs—on social media and panel discussions, at bookstores and colleges, in interviews—arguably more than any writer of literary fiction my age. In 2011, I cofounded MDMAfilms; in 2012, *Vice* published my column Drug-Related Photoshop Art; in 2013, *Rolling Stone* profiled me—"A New Kind of Linsanity"—focusing on my drug use, and the *New York Times* published reviews of *Taipei* titled "The Agony of Ecstasy" and "A Literary Mind, Under the Spell of Drugs and a MacBook"; and in 2014, *Vice* published my McKenna column, the DMT post of which, in May 2016, was the second Google result for DMT. So if the CIA, which had more than twenty thousand employees in 2015, were to track one person in the literary world, it conceivably could be me, I had sometimes, mostly with amusement, imagined. They'd infiltrated a mushroom-seeking trip to Mexico in the 1950s and dosed people with LSD in the 1960s, I knew, and I knew I knew little about the CIA.

Tracy's internet presence, which seemed too original and project-like to be real, as if it were the enjoyably crafted work of a polymathic CIA agent, supported this theory, which had an auspicious inflection. The concrete nightmare of it sometimes resolved, briefly and surprisingly, into a bizarre reality of being with Tracy forever in a performance-art-like existence, forcing me to creatively use all of myself: I believed, for maybe a total of around a minute, that my goal now was to charm and endear Tracy into increasing amounts of interest in my activities, so that, instead of incriminating me, she would let me live my life in my room and just continue to observe me from a distance—that she *was* faking an interest in psychedelics, but my life would now busily and meaningfully, as my only hope to remain free, consist of persuading her to really be interested. I imagined her becoming an intimate, internalized friend who I'd communicate with only indirectly, through the medium of her CIA job.

- A person who hated me. Someone who independently wanted me to go to jail and who, in order to successfully infiltrate my life—to make it into my room and poison, frame, and/or kill me—had gone as far as faking an interest in Terence McKenna and attending an out-of-state psychedelics conference three years in a row. In the past two years, since my computer-disposing trip in August 2013, it had been difficult to enter my life. Focusing on my recovery, I'd indulged the hermit parts of me and stayed alone most of the time, making no effort to be social and negative effort in meeting anyone new or in person. But Tracy had done it, had gotten as far as helping me tape together the device I'd used to smoke what I'd believed was DMT.

Of the four or five theories that I believed for varying amounts of time, this one demoralized and frustrated me most—that a stranger had tracked me online for almost a decade, pounced on my McKenna interest, emailed me to reveal an interest in psychedelics, offered me plant-extracted DMT that she knew I wouldn't refuse, and then, while busy with her own life, framed me for crimes in my own room. Unlike the CIA theory, this one didn't bend into desirability but remained terrible and stinging.

Nine minutes into the second video, the weighty, wood-handled knife was on the floor between Tracy (on the sofa) and me (on the floor around five feet away). In a tone meant to vaguely criticize her apparent massive amount of free time allowing her, as a person who hated me, to track me for years, I'd accusatorily asked her how she made money. Terrified she was going to grab the knife and stab me, I frantically and abruptly, without looking at my hands but continuing to hold eye contact with a blurry Tracy, who was answering my question, snatched and threw the knife to my left, across the room.

"What are you doing?" said Tracy, taken aback.

"Getting rid of that," I mumbled.

"Why? What are you doing? Don't throw things."

"I'm just . . . I'm not throwing it, I'm just moving it over there," I said very quietly.

"You won't throw my stuff, right?"

I was silent, terrified.

"Right?" repeated Tracy.

"No," I said, laughing nervously.

"Okay," said Tracy. "Good."

"That was—yeah, that was my," I said in a moderate whisper. "Pipe," I said in a louder whisper, not wanting Tracy to think I'd thrown a knife, at the same time, however, that she said, "You can throw your stuff—just don't throw my stuff."

"I won't throw your stuff," I said.

"I won't steal your pen," said Tracy. "I just sew, I just do it, I make stuff," she said, continuing to answer my question about her financial situation. "And then people give me money for it, which is cool."

After five seconds of silence, I said, "I'm still trying to understand," in a dejected, tired, resigned voice. I was trying to understand how I'd been so thoroughly deceived.

"I know," said Tracy in an understanding voice I half-heard as patronizing and sadistic. She looked distractedly in her bag.

"What are you looking at?" I said in a quietly panicked voice, believing she was getting a weapon or signaling the police, FBI, or CIA to break down my door.

"I don't know, I thought that was mine," she said, indicating the side of the room I'd blindly thrown the knife—in a sideways manner ending possibly with some sliding—and briefly showing me her pipe, a ceramic piece she'd shown me earlier.

"How do . . . you . . . feel?" I said meekly.

"How do I feel? Fine."

"It seems like you're trying . . ."

"What?" said Tracy. "Don't be so suspicious." Minutes later, she said she was going to leave and asked if I was going to be okay. In an email three days later, she would say, "I didn't understand that you really wanted me to stay until you explicitly said 'I need you to stay, I'm having a bad trip.' I thought you wanted me to leave, because you were so suspicious of me, and I couldn't compare your 'normal' self to your DMT self to know what was happening, because I don't know you well."

"No, I'm not going to be okay," I said in a feeble voice.

Tracy said she was going to take one more hit of my cannabis. Around ten minutes later, she was ready to leave again. Her boyfriend, whom I had suspected existed but hadn't known for sure until then, was outside walking around waiting for her. They were staying in Brooklyn while here for the five-day psychedelics conference, and it was getting late. "Any last words?" she said, which made me feel condemned. "I'm sorry I can't hang out for longer. But I also feel like maybe you want to be alone."

I asked why.

After some thought, Tracy said because I was quiet, like I was thinking a lot.

"But that doesn't mean . . . I want to be . . . alone," I said in a nearly inaudible monotone.

"That's true," said Tracy, and began telling me what had happened, that I'd vaporized DMT into a plastic bottle. I listened, enrapt, and sometimes asked questions. We digressed a few times. I told Tracy I thought she'd killed me. She said she hadn't. I said I'd suspected her of poisoning me. She laughed. "Okay," she said at around 10:24 P.M. "I'm going to go."

I was silent.

"Do you feel better now?"

"I feel like we haven't talked . . . we're still talking . . . I feel like . . ." I said.

"Do you want to keep talking? But earlier you said that you just wanted to write."

"I just wanted to . . . write," I whispered. "When earlier?"

"Before you smoked it," said Tracy.

"Yeah, I did say that, but now something's different," I said cautiously.

She called her boyfriend, and then we continued talking. Finally, at around 10:49 P.M., after she'd finished telling me all she remembered—and after we'd tried to discuss what I remembered of the five minutes after smoking, which at that point, besides that I "interacted" with an "alien," was nothing—I began to fully realize the extent of my paranoia. I began to confidently realize, with immense relief and a quiet, humbling joy, that Tracy was not a CIA or FBI agent, undercover officer, journalist, or vigilante and that nothing terrible or even embarrassing or awkward had happened. Tracy was a friend who had brought me DMT and helped me smoke it and—despite my distrustful, mumbly attitude and seemingly antisocial inability to share anything about my experience—stayed, through my time of paranoid despair, to talk until I finally felt better!

"Thanks for staying," I said, feeling deeply grateful.

"You're welcome. So, you took mushrooms and had a bad time?"

"Not a bad time," I said about my psilocybin trip from two and a sixth years ago, which we'd discussed a little before I smoked DMT. "I just . . . cut a lot of my cords and threw away my computer."

Tracy laughed and asked if I'd been upset afterward.

I shook my head no. "I felt really happy."

At 11:15 P.M., after making sure everything made sense to me, Tracy was ready to leave again. I told her I'd been "really paranoid" before and apologized. She laughed and it sounded friendly and comforting. My voice wasn't quiet anymore. I sounded outgoing. She asked if she could fill her bottle with tap water and I offered mineral water and she accepted and said she needed only a little, enough for an hour. I encouraged her to take as much as she wanted. She laughed and thanked me and we walked to my door. "Bye, thank you," I said.

"Bye, Tao. Have a good night."

"Thank you, you too."

My door closed. A minute later, after doing things out of view—which sounded like moving things around—I appeared in the video smiling happily with an alert, focused demeanor. I typed that Tracy had left and that it was 11:18 P.M., then stopped the video at ninety minutes twenty-nine seconds. I closed my eyes and thought about what to type. "Feel like I was mobbed by alien sex, then I forgot it all," I typed. "Now suddenly I remember having sex with an alien and feeling overwhelmed by it. Maybe aliens love sex with me." I was aware of the inadequacy and redundancy of this; I'd already typed about alien sex, I knew, and wasn't adding anything new. I struggled to remember anything worth noting. "When Tracy was texting, I thought police or CIA were going to break into my room," I typed after a while. I was glad to have remembered this; it reminded me how terrified I'd been. I began watching the ninety-minute video. At 11:31 P.M., Tracy texted "Hows it going?" I responded:

Good, thanks. I've been trying/failing to get the video back. I recorded video of us talking after because I was paranoid and thought you were trying to get me to admit I'd done something horrible when I was blacked out, I was interpreting everything you were saying in terms of this for a long time. Thanks for talking to me until I was okay again.

At 12:20 A.M., Tracy texted "Did that go horribly wrong?" I responded:

No. I like how it went. I was so scared and paranoid but then it turned out I was wrong which I feel good about. I interacted with something tremendous seeming but remember nothing, then got paranoid due to not being mentally in control enough I think is what happened. Thank you for the experience, definitely glad it happened.

Tracy asked if I'd recovered the first video. I said I was trying. She said she still couldn't believe I deleted it. We discussed if I'd smoked too much. In *DMT*, Strassman wrote that he asked Stephen Szára if, in the 1950s, he ever gave his volunteers too much DMT. "Yes," said Szára. "They could not remember anything. They could not bring back memories of the experience. The only thing that remained with them was the feeling that something frightening had happened."

At around 12:50 A.M., I finished watching the second video, and at 1:30 A.M., I texted Tracy that I'd recovered the first video. I uploaded it to Vimeo, emailed her the link and password, and began watching it. The time-sensitive, language-resistant, universe-transcending experience of smoked DMT seemed suited to me as a research subject. It used all of me, was the opposite of boring, could be done alone, and involved writing both autobiographically and about unmapped, unacknowledged worlds. Despite the compatibility, my DMT (and psilocybin) trips had remained mostly terrestrial and biography-muddled. After my hedonistic, alien-sex, and "leave society" trips, I'd now had an exploratory trip with a paranoid after-experience that made me forget what I'd explored. All I remembered was (1) the place of self-twirling entities and (2) when Tracy looked like a reptilian, higher-dimensional being.

My experiences had shown I wasn't ready to explore the unknown. Metaphysical exploration seemed like something one could do for a lifetime, passing on knowledge over generations, which was what aboriginals had done. Modern people, like me, in the global culture, seemed handicapped at it, which therefore made it challenging. The activity asked me to be healthier and more patient and self-aware, to have better memory and language skills, to learn, feel, notice, and understand more.

At 3:30 A.M., summarizing my last two hours, I typed "Recovered the video! By deleting a photo, then going to Edit then Undo Delete twice. Then watched it, then returned to beginning and summarized first 19:32 of video, working hard." I was asleep an hour later. "Can close my eyes and enjoyably deeply imagine and hear Chopin sonatas" was the last note I typed, at 4:11 A.M., very stoned, having enjoyed cannabis throughout the late night.

SALVIA

"A new psychedelic has been discovered that is active in the microgram range, exactly as LSD is, but it's not related to LSD at all, nor is it related to any other known psychoactive substance," said McKenna in "The New Psychedelics" (1995) in Amsterdam about salvinorin A. It was news he also shared in other talks that, and the previous, year. "DMT test-pilots come back white-knuckled and ashen from these places," he said about where the 59-atom compound, a dose of which, at 300 micrograms, was the size of a small grain of salt, transported people. Salvinorin A interacted only with κ-opioid and D_2 receptors—unlike psilocin and DMT, which interacted with at least seventeen receptors, or LSD, which interacted with at least twenty-one—and was made by *Salvia divinorum*, a species of sage introduced to modern people in 1961 by the Mazatec, who'd also, in 1938, introduced us to psilocybin mushrooms.

My first time smoking salvia, at night in the Standard Hotel in October 2012 during my "recovery," the only effect I noticed was that my voice seemed to become squeakily high-pitched, but when

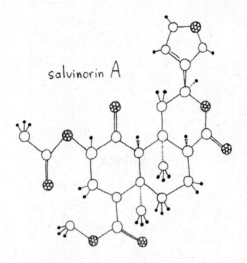

salvinorin A

I asked if I sounded different, my friends seemed to ignore me. Seconds later, Gian smoked salvia and stood and ran out of the room into the hallway because, he explained after returning, he'd felt inside a snake whose scales dropped away behind him as he ran. The second time was sixteen days later, in my room with Gwen and a third person we'd never met—a filmmaker paying us $40 to record us smoking salvia. After smoking, I went to light the pipe for Gwen and, realizing I was trying to do something I'd be hilariously, it seemed, unable to within deciseconds, burst out laughing before going unconscious. The third time, I felt mild, vague effects.

The fourth time was a month after that, in February 2014. Sitting on my bed, I smoked a hit of dried salvia leaf that I'd ordered online, choosing 5x potency from a selection reaching 60x. I lay on my back and noticed that part of the ceiling was extremely distorted, like in a Dalí painting. I calmly thought, "Melting," and "Weird, that's a stereotypical psychedelic thing I've never experienced and didn't think really happened," and "That's not weird then; it just actually happens, interesting." I sat, exhaled, smoked hit 2, lay supine, and closed my eyes.

After a few seconds, I blacked out fully and I think briefly. I was next aware of having convinced myself, while unconscious, to go to the beach. In my thirteen years in New York, I'd never been to the beach. I felt amazed I was going. "Beach," I said in a strange and tinny voice. "I'm going to the beach," I said to somehow, by saying and hearing this, confirm if I was or not. It seemed my body was momentarily going to go all the way to the beach—to Coney Island, I sensed, more than an hour away—and that I wasn't in control. I didn't want to go, but my mind seemed to have been jarred backward one or two seconds, or somehow laterally, moving it beyond where it could control my body. When I saw *Being John Malkovich* (1999) in college, I enjoyed its deadpan tone and absurd world, in which a portal existed in a building in Manhattan that led to the inside perspective of John Malkovich. Now I felt inside myself in a *Being John Malkovich* manner, disconnected and trapped. My only role now seemed to be to observe. Passively observing my life had seemed attractive to me in the past—I'd described it in fiction as a pleasant-seeming state—but I hadn't taken into account that, as I realized then with dread and panic, I wouldn't only observe but would also feel whatever happened. I sensed my body would behave "out of character" at the beach and, on other days, elsewhere and that I would feel anxiety, tedium, shame, and discomfort. I sat, stood, and—around half a minute, I estimate, after hit 2—walked two or three steps toward my front door before I was able to stop myself from going. Relieved, I lay on my bed, closed my eyes, and immediately forgot about the beach.

To my surprise, my entire weight felt precariously supported on a fence exactly aligned with my spine. This entranced me for minutes. Then I felt like I was being vaguely scooped by a bulldozer in a reddish, dusty, skyless, barren landscape. Sometimes

I was a scooper, dragging harshly against concrete. My expectation that this feel painful and abrasive inflected some original sensation into what I felt: physically awkward in a complicatedly pleasing, unfamiliarly texture-related, fascinating manner. At one point my tongue felt like a building-size slab of concrete, powerfully scraping an unseen surface far below. At another point I was the slab, being invisibly dragged at an angle like a falling domino with other massive slabs. My motion seemed extradimensionally controlled, which made me feel like I was inside a computer game. I sensed roughness and danger, the possibility of things being crushed, but the situation felt productive and somewhat peaceful, like a construction site. At times, I felt less like a consciousness in this world than the world itself, focused on a specific scene in the universe of me. I sensed how on a larger dose I could completely enter this world.

Near the end of the trip and lingeringly afterward, supine on my bed, I felt that entities as different to me as I am to a cloud or lake could and were, in their way that I couldn't comprehend so wasn't bothered by, observing me. The building I was in—densely packed with six floors of walls—seemed somewhat comically to not conceal anything. I felt more in the sky, outer space, and hyperspace than in a building. At 3:49 P.M., thirty-two minutes after hit 1, I began typing the first draft of this account of my fourth time smoking salvia. It was February 25, 2014, seventeen months after I encountered McKenna, and I hadn't encountered the information in the rest of this chapter.

KATHLEEN HARRISON

In "Indigenous Plant Wisdom" (2001), a talk in Palenque, Mexico, Kathleen LaPriel Harrison shared something she did a month prior, in December 2000, at a salvia conference in Oregon. After declining on joining, she'd agreed to watch over seven people as they ate salvia leaves in an octagonal room late at night. Thirteen had shown—"and that was okay," said Harrison, who in 2013 would estimate that 60 percent of her experiences with "different medicines" had been solitary and comment "that's the kind of 'investigator' I am." She used the opportunity to try an idea she got from the Mazatec—that everyone pray together in soft voices. The group created a "tapestry of sound, rolling" then ate the leaves. "And then one person had that occasional experience, that thing that you hear of with usually the stronger salvinorin kind of doses, of suddenly wanting to bolt!" For forty minutes, quietly because everyone had agreed on silence, Harrison prevented the "very strong little dude" from going outside where there was snow. She learned a lot—about containing energy, cajoling, whispering—that night, she said in her Palenque talk, which included slides.

One slide showed the male and female flowers of corn. "I just wanted to be sure that we understand that sacred plants bridge many categories," said Harrison. She explained that she taught part-time at a university and also talked to the herbal community, including to native plant societies, and that the way she discussed psychoactive plants "in the so-called 'straight world'" was by embedding them within the entire spectrum of plants used by humans. "And there is a way that we can infiltrate, lovingly and effectively," she said, and laughed. "And I don't mean infiltrate—you know, kind of joking, but—I just think that we overcategorize, so I try to embed it. So, therefore, corn is a sacred plant, there you go," she said, and showed the next slide.

In her Palenque talk, in January 2001 at the Entheobotany Conference, Harrison also shared her history with the Mazatec. Around seven years earlier, she decided to go to them. She'd grown up in the 1950s on the Californian Channel Islands—where her naturalist dad taught her to pay attention to nature—and had visited Mexico when she was six, spending months in a small village, and then throughout her life, including a six-month trip in 1973 and 1974, but she'd never visited the Mazatec. She talked to her friend Bret Blosser—who'd chewed thirteen pairs of salvia leaves in a Mazatec ceremony in the mid-1980s and found himself "out of the three dimensions and linear time"—and he introduced her to a shamanic Mazatec family.

Harrison had visited the Mazatec three times and was going again after the conference. Staying five or six weeks per trip, she immersed herself in their worldview by helping them harvest crops, clean beans, and watch grandchildren; by listening to conversations, collecting plants, playing with children, and taking photographs; and by sleeping on their floors and also in a rented place of her own, where she could write.

THE MAZATEC

In 2016, there were 7,080 million modern people in 196 countries and, the UN estimated, 370 million aboriginal people in 5,000 groups, at least 62 of which lived in Mexico, including 16 in Oaxaca, one of which, inhabiting the Sierra Mazateca since an unknown period of time before the Spanish arrived in the sixteenth century, was the Mazatec. In "Roads Where There Have Long Been Trails" (1998), an essay about her time with the Mazatec, Harrison quoted a Zapotec man from another part of Oaxaca: "My people know many herbs; so do the Mixtec and the Mixe. But the Mazatecs know magic. They know how the plants talk."

In "Spirit in Nature: Psychedelic Plants and Mushrooms Through Native Eyes" (2008), Harrison described the Mazatec as "kind of self-isolating," keeping to themselves not only from other linguistic groups but also from one another. When she began her fieldwork with the Mazatec in 1994, around 40 percent of them spoke only their own language, which had many dialects, even after five hundred years of colonization, which meant, observed Harrison, that "an equivalent amount of their knowledge, their lore, their stories, their songs, and probably their information about the natural world" was intact. Among the psychoactive plants and fungi used by the Mazatec were two species of morning glory (also used in childbirth), many species of psilocybin mushrooms (called "the little ones that spring forth," "the little holy children," "the landslide," and other folk names), and *Salvia divinorum*, which once grew only where they lived.

Harrison said many people had "just plain weird" and some had "bad" experiences with the plant and that she felt this was due to how it was used, then shared what she'd learned from the Mazatec, the only known people with a tradition of using it.

- The plant grew in filtered light "in little glades in the woods" and liked to be moist and cool. "They always refer to it as her, and I try to do that too," said Harrison. "She's very shy. She's very powerful, but she's very shy." The Mazatec grew her off the trail to keep her clean. They compared her to the deer, which are startled away by noise or quick movements.

- Harrison waited years before telling them salvia had gotten out and people were smoking the dried leaves. They were appalled by the drying, doubly appalled by the smoking. "That won't work—that will just really offend her," Harrison said they said. "She won't show up. Whatever you're getting it's not her."

- The Mazatec ate salvia in pitch dark—rolled-up wilted leaves "like a large salad rolled into a cigar." Before the experience, they stated their intentions, which they returned to throughout in "a kind of murmuring prayer." They did not do it to "see what will happen." They did it asking for help, a gift, or a favor.

- They said not to do it alone. Sitting close, they guarded the person doing it because of "the bolt factor"—that around 10 percent get up and start moving and later don't remember what they did.

- They said not to laugh because laughter scares away the spirit of the plant. "People have experienced salvia as being something that gives them the uncontrollable giggles," said Harrison, and shared an example: She knew a Buddhist who fell "passionately in love" with a toaster after smoking salvia. "And that so amused him that he found himself rolling on the ground laughing. And when he came out of it he was just like, 'I've been a Buddhist monk for decades—what *happened* to me?'"

Which reminded me of the fifth—and most recent—time I smoked salvia. On my sofa in my room, in July 2014, I became aware of myself talking to my bong. When I realized I was earnestly asking my bong for advice on what to do about feeling lonely, I said, "The bong can't tell you," aloud in a playfully scolding tone, then laughed hysterically for a while.

Harrison called the toaster experience "amusing" and "even interesting" but said it wasn't what she was after, personally. She desired a relationship with the species's spirit. She was "fascinated by their worldviews," but fascination wasn't the main reason she directed her attention to the Mazatec and other aboriginals. It was because she felt that, after doing it for so long, they'd figured out the spiritual and behavioral technology of relating to *Salvia divinorum* and other species in order to get "the best result," which she defined as "the most rebalancing of oneself" so that one could "do work in the world that is balancing also."

THE EDGE OF THE GARDEN

Sisters of the Extreme: Women Writing on the Drug Experience, the retitled, expanded second edition of *Shaman Woman, Mainline Lady* (1982), was published in 2000 by Park Street Press. The anthology had eighty-seven contributors, including George Sand on opium, Anaïs Nin and Julie Doucet on LSD, Alice B. Toklas and Maya Angelou on cannabis, Valentina Wasson on psilocybin, Ann Shulgin on MDMA, and—one of the additions—Kathleen Harrison on salvia.

In "The Leaves of the Shepherdess," Harrison wrote about her heart, which had always murmured but began beating irregularly in a more disturbing manner after her divorce and the death of her dad. Harrison saw a doctor, then decided to travel to Mexico to ask a Mazatec healer to do a ceremony for her with the Leaves of the Shepherdess. "The curandero unrolled banana-leaf bundles of hand-sized *Salvia divinorum* leaves, slightly wilted, and sorted them into pairs," wrote Harrison, who received forty pairs, representing feminine and masculine, rolled into "a long wad." She was told not to hesitate at their bitterness, stop until she'd eaten them all, or laugh. "Suddenly there was a shimmering, the curandero blew the candles out for total darkness, and within seconds I was completely in another realm, astonished. Some part of me ate the final bite and I relaxed into another place: I was in the presence of a great female being, a woman, twenty feet high and semitransparent."

In a talk in 2010, Harrison said the Mazatec had been engaged for probably millennia in "profound psychedelic investigations" in order to cure, to invoke and exchange with "forces and deities," and to ask the questions "What is it all about, really?" and "What *is* real?"

Harrison realized she couldn't move her feet. She felt the *curandero*, his wife, his son, and "the little granddaughter" giving the spirit their full attention. They were plants at the edge of the spirit's garden. The spirit's hand passed through Harrison's chest twice and "a pocket of hurt blew away." Returning to the present, Harrison heard "Show them the edge of the garden" repeatedly in Spanish and English. "That is my work," ended her essay.

FROM THE GODDESS

The age of the Mazatec–salvia relationship is unknown. If salvia and pipiltzintzintli—a plant used by the Aztecs, who also used psilocybin mushrooms, peyote, and daturas and who gave the Mazatec their name, which means "the deer people"—are the same, as R. Gordon Wasson theorized, the relationship could be at least seven hundred years old. If salvia is pipiltzintzintli, it probably once grew over a much larger area than its "current, extremely limited distribution," said a 2010 paper that identified *Salvia venulosa*—a species that did not make salvinorin A and was known from only three locations in the Colombian Andes—as *Salvia divinorum*'s closest relative. If salvia is not pipiltzintzintli, maybe the relationship is somehow only one hundred to four hundred years old; that the Mazatec name for the plant, Shka Maria Pastora, has two Spanish words serves as evidence for this mysterious possibility, about which McKenna, in one talk, theorizing on the "puzzlement," said, "I think it is sent from the Goddess at this time."

Whatever its age and origins, *Salvia divinorum* was once, for at least centuries, before a specimen was brought to UCLA's Botanical Garden in 1962, limited to the cloud forests of the Sierra Mazateca, but now, through cloning (growing cuttings into single-parent plants), lived in homes and gardens worldwide. "It is speculated that the species diminished its ability to set seed through centuries of human tending," wrote Harrison in 2000. "And perhaps this highly sensitive species—growing in light-speckled seclusion in such a small region of the world—would have long ago disappeared, had it not been for its lovely *medicina* and gift to human consciousness."

In May 2016, a PhD thesis by Ivan Casselman at Southern Cross Plant Science revealed that *Salvia divinorum* makes rosmarinic acid, a 42-atom compound with antioxidant, anti-inflammatory, anti-depression, anti-bacterial, and anti-viral properties that treated herpes simplex, had potential in treating Alzheimer's, and was common in the Lamiaceae, or mint, family. Casselman cited eight studies from 2000 to 2011 that found salvia and/or salvinorin A had low toxicity. He suggested the plant be "recognized as a threatened species" due to low genetic variation and population, and observed that the Mazatec, of which around three hundred thousand existed, also used the plant to treat diarrhea, headaches, rheumatism, and a Mazatec illness called "swollen belly" that was caused by being cursed.

THE SALVIA VIDEOS

Starting in 2002 with Australia and 2005 with Missouri, countries and states began to criminalize *Salvia divinorum*. The species and its unique compound joined psilocybin, DMT, LSD, and other psychedelics as illegal for use in scientific research, self-help, art, psychotherapy, solving problems, disrupting addictions, catalyzing change, and other practices and activities. On November 27, 2006, when salvia was regulated in five states, KSL-TV in Salt Lake City aired an "Eyewitness Investigation" titled "Dangerous Herb Is Legal in Utah" that showed a young man named Jim laughing and saying, "I feel like the octopus ride" after smoking salvia. Reporter Debbie Dujanovic brought videos of people smoking salvia to a high school football game on a DVD, showed parents, and had this conversation:

DUJANOVIC: The herb is called salvia. Have you heard of it?
DAD: No, never heard of that.
DUJANOVIC: Detectives we've talked to say it gives kids the same high as LSD.
MOM: Really. I've never even heard of it.
DUJANOVIC: What do you think?
MOM: And children here are using this? That can't be right for it to be legal.
DAD: That should be illegal.

The next night on KSL-TV, in "Lawmaker Responds to Investigative Report on Dangerous Herb," Dujanovic reported on the previous night's investigation. "Moments after our story ended, Utah Representative Paul Ray began writing a bill to ban salvia," she said, commending the lawmaker's frantic haste. A local police department, she added, was "also reacting," had decided to "educate officers about the herb." Ray himself said three sentences in the brief segment: "It was upsetting to see we have a drug of that strength that's legal. We're basically going to make it illegal to possess or sell. Period."

On June 10, 2008, "Writing a Letter to Congress on Salvia" was uploaded to YouTube. In the video, Erik Hoffstad smoked salvia on a sofa and tried to write a letter to Paul Ray, who after a year and a half had failed to regulate the plant. Hoffstad laughed intensely and deeply and satisfyingly, it seemed to me, for 55 of the video's 180 seconds, making me smile and grin and also laugh. In another video, uploaded sixteen days earlier, he'd tried to garden on salvia. The two videos, among the most-watched salvia videos on YouTube—a website that started in April 2005—with 1.8 and 2.2 million views after eight years, showed him unable to do the physical tasks in a manner indicating he'd left concrete reality; they, and other salvia videos in which stationary people have facial expressions conveying they're conscious elsewhere, experiencing awe, reminded me that, using only plants and fungi that have evolved over millions of years and been selected and used by humans over millennia, I can safely travel to the furthest places humans have gone and stay there 5 or 30 or 120 minutes, during which I can experientially research consciousness, death, time, existence, magic, ecstasy, and the mystery within a tradition older than agriculture.

Three months after Hoffstad's videos, when salvia was regulated in thirteen states, including Florida, where possession was punishable by five years in prison, the *New York Times* published a front-page article that began "With a friend videotaping, 27-year-old Christopher Lenzini of Dallas took a hit of *Salvia divinorum*, regarded as the world's most potent hallucinogenic herb, and soon began to imagine, he said, that he was in a boat with little green men." The article reported that the "rare claims of salvia-related deaths" (two suicides blamed on salvia) had been "speculative"; that "salvia-related emergency room admissions" were "virtually nonexistent" even though 1.8 million people, according to the government, had tried it; that in many states "the YouTube videos" had become "Exhibit A in legislative efforts to regulate salvia"; and that pharmacologists who felt salvia could treat addiction, depression, and pain feared its criminalization would make it hard to do tests on humans.

Six years later, in 2014, the Associated Press published an article about Paul Ray, who'd continued failing to ban *Salvia divinorum* and seemed to have stopped trying, titled "Utah Lawmaker Proposes Bringing Back Firing Squads for Executions." The next year, Utah became one of the two states where execution—a punishment illegal in around 60 percent of countries—by firing squad was legal, reversing its 2004 banning of the method. A year later, in 2016, salvia remained legal in Utah but was illegal to some degree in around 14 percent of countries and at least 62 percent of states. In twenty-one states it was a Schedule I drug.

WHY ARE PSYCHEDELICS ILLEGAL?

On March 1, 2016, in the morning, I rode an elevator to the eleventh floor of a building in Chinatown and sat in a surprisingly high-ceilinged—for being so far up in the sky—courtroom with sixty to eighty people. Two grand juries, we learned, would be selected that day. Those not chosen could go home; the rest would begin their service. The 60 to 70 percent of us, it seemed by a show of hands, who'd deferred thrice could not, it was explained, get out of jury duty again; if our name was called, we had to say "serve" and go sit with the other chosen ones. Using a hand-operated, lottery-seeming, plastic ball filled with folded paper, a man called out forty-six names in an impressively subtle, game-show-like voice that amused me and others in, I felt, a calming manner. With twenty-two other people who lived in Manhattan, I was selected for a "special narcotics" grand jury, which meant we'd hear mostly only drug cases.

I'd deferred three times in two years and now—thirteen days after I began writing this book—had been selected to serve on a rare, drug-focused grand jury. I viewed this coincidence as a gift for my drug-focused book to absorb.

We rode the elevator down, crossed the street into another building, rode an elevator up, entered a small courtroom, and sat where we'd sit the rest of the day and for nine more days. I was stoned, not abnormally, on baked cannabis. We received the 2015 edition of *Grand Juror's Handbook*, which said only 29,000, or around 5 percent, of the 574,000 jurors in New York in 2005 were grand jurors; the rest were trial jurors. We watched videos that seemed, to me, surreal and sometimes surprisingly funny. I began, after around an hour, falling asleep. Others seemed to also struggle, in the large, soft seats, to stay awake. After a lunch break, we watched more videos. Four times during this second session of videos, I laughed uncontrollably for seconds while no one else was laughing but seemingly without attracting attention—probably because my laughter was quiet and involved little to no movement. After the videos, there was time to hear a case.

We learned from two officers that they'd bought drugs from someone—the accused person—while undercover, working on a team that did this regularly. Then it was time to vote.

For each charge, we'd vote to indict or dismiss. According to our handbooks, people couldn't be brought to trial for a felony unless they'd been "indicted by a grand jury." We voted to indict weapon and cocaine charges but not a charge for marijuana. Then we voted on if we wanted to deliberate. More than eleven raised their hands, so the deliberation began.

Someone in back asked why we dismissed marijuana but indicted "a dinky pocketknife." He spoke in a manner that seemed designed to influence jurors to also dismiss the weapon charge but which, I felt, could be interpreted to mean he felt we should not have dismissed the marijuana charge.

The juror to my left, either having the latter interpretation or just taking the opportunity to defend marijuana, said because marijuana—the court's name for cannabis—had never killed anyone. One or two others spoke—we acknowledged that, obviously, we should have deliberated *before* voting—and then the deliberation, and day 1, ended.

The words "marihuana" and "marijuana" became popular in the 1930s, when newspapers published headlines like, in 1933, "Murder Weed Found Up and Down Coast—Deadly Marihuana Dope Plant Ready for Harvest That Means Enslavement of California Children," and when Henry Anslinger, the first commissioner of the Federal Bureau of Narcotics, which was founded in 1930 when cannabis was banned in twenty-four states, "depicted marijuana as a sinister substance that made Mexican and African American men lust after white women," wrote Martin A. Lee in *Smoke Signals* (2012). Anslinger avoided the word "cannabis" because few people "knew that marijuana, the weed that some blacks and Chicanos were smoking, was merely a weaker version of the concentrated cannabis medicines that everyone had been taking since childhood," wrote Lee. In 1937, when cannabis, which comes from the Greek *kánnabis*, a word at least 2,500 years old, was banned in thirty-five states, the Marihuana Tax Act was passed, making possession illegal federally. At the congressional hearing for the act, which he co-drafted, Anslinger said these sentences:

- This drug is as old as civilization itself.

- We seem to have adopted the Mexican terminology, and we call it marihuana, which means good feeling.

- In India it is sold over the counter to the addicts, direct, and there it is known as "bhang" and "ganja."

- It is impossible to say what the effect will be on any individual.

- It is dangerous to the mind and body, and particularly dangerous to the criminal type, because it releases all of the inhibitions.

- Not long ago we found a fifteen-year-old boy going insane because, the doctor told the enforcement officers, he thought the boy was smoking marihuana cigarettes.

- Last year the state of Pennsylvania destroyed two hundred thousand pounds.

- We have always pointed the finger of scorn at China, and now marihuana is being smuggled out to China, by sailors.

- It makes very fine cordage, and this legislation exempts the mature stalk when it is grown for hemp purposes.

Anslinger—who was head of the FBN until retiring in 1962, six years before the FBN merged with the BDAC to form the BNDD, which in 1973 merged with the ODALE to become the DEA—continued being both informative and inaccurate in material submitted for the public record of the hearing, writing, among other sentences:

- The plant was known by the Greeks as "nepenthe" and was lauded in the immortal Odyssey of Homer.

- In the argot of the underworld it has colloquial, colorful names such as "reefer," "muggles," "Indian hay," "hot hay," and "weed."

- Its use frequently leads to insanity.

The term "420" originated "among California teenagers in the 1970s," wrote Chris Duvall in *Cannabis* (2015), which was published in the UK. Duvall described the "internationally important" code word as "the number '420'—pronounced 'four-twenty', and including the time '4:20' and the American-style date '4/20'." He wrote: "Even the authorities take notice: on 20 April 2006, the U.S. Food and Drug Administration reiterated its view that drug *Cannabis* is medically useless."

On day 2, we heard six or seven cases. Each case began with the judge and his assistant leaving the room; a stenographer entering and sitting at a typewriter with large, rubber buttons; and a prosecutor entering and saying the name of the accused person, the charges, the witnesses, and if we'd see any evidence, like photos and/or videos, then leaving and returning with the first witness. In one of the cases we heard that morning—which I share as a representative case—the prosecutor left and returned with a police officer, who seemed to be in his late twenties. Juror 2, our "foreperson," asked if the officer swore to tell the truth, "so help you God." He did. He sat in the booth.

The prosecutor asked him questions and we learned that he'd bought three "twists" of crack from the accused person, who we knew only by name. The prosecutor's job was to mediate our interactions with the witnesses, who, it seemed, could only

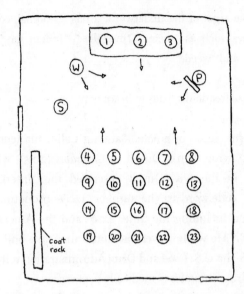

respond to questions. The prosecutor asked if we had further questions. We didn't.

The second witness—the first's commanding officer—was called. We learned from him that the first witness had brought him drugs, which he'd confirmed via field test was crack cocaine, which he'd vouchered, after which he'd filled out a form, which we saw projected on a screen. The prosecutor asked the officer to explain how the test worked and he did.

The prosecutor asked if we had questions. At least two jurors, including me, raised their hands. The prosecutor walked to Juror 12, who asked the prosecutor—in, as we'd been instructed, a quiet voice—to ask the officer if he'd tested all three twists. The prosecutor returned to the podium, asked the question. The officer said he'd tested only one. The prosecutor looked at Juror 12, who raised his hand. The prosecutor walked to him, conferred quietly, returned to the podium, asked why. The officer said there was no reason why—they just did it that way. I laughed a little.

The prosecutor walked to me, Juror 5.

"How did he learn of the defendant?" I said quietly.

The prosecutor seemed confused.

"How did he learn of the defendant?"

After a second, the prosecutor said, "Right," returned to the podium, and asked the officer how he learned of the accused person. When the accused person was brought to him by the first witness in handcuffs, answered the officer. The prosecutor looked at me, walked to me, leaned toward me. I asked how the first officer, who bought the drugs, learned of the accused person. I was curious. Poor minorities seemed more likely to be targeted than, say, college students living in dorms.

In "Legalize It All," a "report" in the April 2016 issue of *Harper's*, Dan Baum shared something the assistant to the president for Domestic Affairs under Richard Nixon told him in 1994: "The Nixon campaign in 1968, and the Nixon White House after that, had two enemies: the antiwar left and black people. You understand what I'm saying? We knew we couldn't make it illegal to be either against the war or black, but by getting the public to associate the hippies with marijuana and blacks with heroin, and then criminalizing both heavily, we could disrupt those communities."

"He isn't going to be able to tell you that," said the prosecutor.

I laughed in an unself-conscious, jolly-sounding manner. "Oh, right," I said smiling. People continued to seem unbothered by my laughter. What to me was increased laughter just brought me up, I felt, to the level of a normally—or somewhat above-averagely—good-humored, not-grim person. Cannabis did this to me, for which I was grateful.

Two more jurors asked questions, then the witness, prosecutor, and stenographer left and we voted on if we wanted to deliberate. Fewer than twelve did, so we moved on to the crack-selling charge. Fifteen voted to indict. Due to the seating arrangement, all twenty-two other jurors could see my vote, but I could see only six other votes—unless I turned around, which I didn't except once or twice slightly, allowing me to see eight or nine votes—and all were to indict. Fifteen exceeded eleven, so the person who'd allegedly sold crack and was currently in a cell, where he could be held for forty-five days, would now go on trial to learn his punishment.

The Controlled Substances Act of 1970 differentiated "drugs, substances, or chemicals"—or "drugs"—into five schedules. Drugs with psychedelic—or, in the government's preferred terminology, "hallucinogenic"—effects were Schedule I, which meant they had "no currently accepted medical use and a high potential for abuse." The Drug Enforcement Administration formed in 1973, under Nixon, to enforce the act. Of the six examples of Schedule I drugs on the DEA's website in 2017—

> heroin, lysergic acid diethylamide (LSD), marijuana (cannabis), 3,4-methylenedioxymethamphetamine (ecstasy), methaqualone, and peyote

—three were psychedelic (LSD, cannabis, peyote), two were plants (cannabis, peyote), at least four and arguably all had medical use, and only one (methaqualone) was made by corporations but not since 1985 due to hundreds of deaths. By listing three psychedelics and avoiding more than one representative from any other class of drug, the DEA seemed to strongly convey that psychedelics were the most useless and destructive class of drugs, which has been the opposite of my experience. None of the DEA's examples of Schedule IV drugs ("low potential for abuse and low risk of dependence") was psychedelic, growable, or natural; all were sold by corporations—

Xanax, Soma, Darvon, Darvocet, Valium, Ativan, Talwin, Ambien, Tramadol

—and the DEA refrained from including any chemical names, sharing only the selling-and-advertising-optimized, capitalized brand names. The DEA listed nine examples, as if to squeeze in more for promotional purposes. Seven were opioids or benzodiazepines—two of the three classes of drugs with, I feel based on experience, the most potential for self-destruction and highest risk of dependence (the third being amphetamines, which are Schedule II), an opinion supported by statistics: In 2016, the *New York Times* reported there were 43,982 drug overdose deaths in 2013—none from psilocybin, DMT, salvia, LSD, or cannabis—including 22,767 from prescription drugs, with 16,235 and 6,973 involving opioids and benzodiazepines.

"I don't live there, no," I emailed my mom at 6:04 A.M. on day 3, which was March 3. I'd been waking early to work on this book's first three chapters. "I just go to a courtroom on the 6th floor each day from 10 A.M. to around 4:20 P.M. We have a 1-hour lunch break and 3–4 other breaks." I told my mom I was "voting 'no' for every case" because I felt it was "a waste of time and money to pursue these drug cases" and that, whenever the drug was marijuana, a "slight majority" of jurors voted no.

At around 11:00 A.M. that day, we heard our only non-drug case, which had our only non-officer witness—a low-level employee of a college. We learned a student had paid off his student loans in three transfers over two or three months totaling around $140,000 from the college itself back to the loan company, five years earlier. The witness didn't know exactly how this was achieved but assured us the flaw in the system allowing the felony had been fixed.

We seemed bolder with this case than the drug cases because, I think, for most jurors it probably seemed offensive, unseemly, or incomprehensible—or like it might appear so to others—to question officers when it was officers against drug dealers. We asked six or seven questions, which wasn't enough to learn where the accused person was currently. In custody? Enjoying life with a college degree thinking he'd gotten away with it? Thirteen jurors voted to indict.

A major reason psychedelics are illegal seems to be because of the increasing influence, in the twentieth and twenty-first centuries, of corporations, which are existentially required to increase both revenue and profits in a reliable, competitive, continual manner because their sole function is to grow in value so that their stockholders will own more valuable stock.

Corporations have existed for only around 450 years or 0.16 percent of the time since *Homo sapiens* evolved. I learned about them as a child because the first two medical laser companies my dad founded went public, or became corporations, when I was in elementary and high school, in 1991 and 1999, and because my parents became obsessed with the stock market when I was a child and for years I'd been interested also, reading penny stock message boards and investing my parents' money. Publicly owned companies—the term I prefer because it puts the blame more accurately on everyone—either grow or quickly shrink

and vanish. They don't grow to a certain size and begin divert-
ing profits to workers and carefully ensuring they aren't harming
the planet, their customers, and future and unsuspecting life-
forms—not because they're evil, or because they don't want to,
but because this option isn't available to them as it is for privately
owned companies. Publicly owned companies can survive only
by constantly growing and so their only choice is to automatically
and mindlessly—through the decisions of boards of people representing the stockholders, or investors, who decentrally own the
company—slough off CEOs, CFOs, and other employees who
aren't helping the stock price significantly increase, meaning that
opposing employees of corporations, or supporting one corpora-
tion over another, has no effect on the metaphysical entity called
"corporations."

The pharmaceutical drug industry—whose ten largest companies, all publicly owned, earned around $440 billion in revenue
in 2014, when global revenue of legal drugs exceeded $1 trillion
for the first time—would lose probably tens to, eventually, hundreds of billions of dollars annually if psychedelics became legal,
because hundreds of millions of people could then cheaply and
effectively and sustainably, instead of expensively, ineffectively,
toxically, and fatally, relieve and/or treat depression, anxiety,
addiction, pain, inflammation, insomnia, nausea, thanatopho-
bia, epilepsy, cancer, asthma, dementia, arthritis, fibromyalgia,
cluster headaches, PTSD, OCD, ADHD, Tourette, and other problems with cannabis, psilocybin, DMT, salvia, LSD, mescaline,
and ibogaine, as users of psychedelics have known or suspected
for millennia, aboriginals have known for tens to hundreds of
millennia, and science has begun to confirm since the fifties in
two main waves of research, the second beginning in 2006 at
Johns Hopkins and New York University.

———

By day 4, we were, on many charges, not getting enough votes to either indict or dismiss. Fewer of us were raising our hands to indict cannabis, weapons (mostly knives), paraphernalia (scales, plastic baggies), and possession charges. Since most cases also involved cocaine, crack, and/or heroin—which we seemed to view as obviously unforgivable—our dismissals were relatively insubstantial, punishment-wise. Selling—or having and intending to sell—up to 28 grams of "a mixture containing crack" was punishable, for example, by up to twenty years in jail and $1 million, I learned online. In the courtroom, we weren't told punishments because that was for the trial jury to decide. Our job was to indict or dismiss. With each charge, we first voted to indict; if fewer than twelve raised their hands, we voted to dismiss. If fewer than twelve raised their hands, the charge remained undefined and the prosecutor could ask us to vote again later or bring the case to another grand jury.

Another reason psychedelics have been globally illegal for almost five decades is, I feel, because most people, not surprisingly, believe they are, in addition to pointless and frivolous, very dangerous. McKenna stressed the remarkably benign nature of the substances he promoted—sometimes by comparison to alcohol, cigarettes, sugar, cocaine, caffeine, and even MDMA and ketamine, which he observed hadn't been user-tested for millennia. He specifically advocated natural substances—psilocybin, DMT, salvia, cannabis, ayahuasca—he'd determined to be safe in the short- and long-term. In "Psychedelics Before and After History" (1987), he shared "three tests to apply to a compound that you're thinking of ingesting."

- Does it come from a plant or fungus? ("Plants are also biological systems like us, they cannot produce truly alien compounds.")

- Does it have a history of shamanic usage? ("If a compound is toxic, triggers psychosis, is mutagenic, or induces tumors, it will have been dropped long ago by human groups who experiment with these things.")

- Does it have an affinity to brain chemistry? ("If you take a drug and the next day you feel lousy, and the next day you sort of feel okay, that's not a very good drug; that's an insult to the physical brain.")

He said it was "probably okay to go ahead" if a drug passed at least two tests. "This is a task of a lifetime, so you want compounds which are extremely effective in delivering the noetic experience, the plunge into the tremendum, but you also want to be able to race again another day," he said. Yet his *New York Times* obituary, published in 2000, was able to say he advocated "substances that many experts consider highly dangerous." Three paragraphs later, after quoting a fragment of praise from Jerry Garcia, calling McKenna "the only person who has made a serious effort to objectify the psychedelic experience," the obituary referenced experts again—"But experts on drug treatment attacked Mr. McKenna for popularizing dangerous substances"—and quoted a letter by Judy Corman, vice president of a drug treatment center:

Surely the fact that Terence McKenna says that the psilocybin mushroom "is the megaphone used by an alien, intergalactic Other to communicate with mankind" is enough for us to wonder if taking LSD has done something to his mental faculties.

Corman's letter, which the *New York Times* had published on May 9, 1993, misleadingly quoted not McKenna himself but, I learned, a May 2, 1993, *New York Times* profile of McKenna that said, "One thing he argues is that the psilocybin mushroom, Stropharia cubensis, is no ordinary life form, no lowly fungus, but in fact the megaphone used by an alien, intergalactic Other to communicate with mankind." Corman's letter cited multiple deaths of athletes from cocaine and argued, "Whether it's LSD, marijuana, cocaine or heroin, the message from *The Times* should clearly be that drug abuse is dangerous."

On day 5, when we heard no cases, a juror asked me if I was the writer Tao Lin. As part of me considered if there was a way I could say no, I said yes. She, a woman in her thirties, Juror 11, said her sister was a fan of my writing. She asked if I was going to write about my jury experience. I said I wrote, in some way, in notes or books, about almost everything I did, so probably yes. I said I felt the student who paid off his student loans with his college's money shouldn't have been punished, and she laughed. I felt comfortable saying this because I'd noticed that she and Juror 12 were the two most question-asking jurors—the two most involved and unautomatic in their judgments and who most wanted, it seemed, to deliberate.

That night, in my room, to amuse myself, I imagined Juror 11 was a CIA agent. I also spent minutes thinking about my "CIA novel," a novel about an autobiographical writer who suspects various people of working for the CIA, which I enjoyed fantasizing about writing. At this point, on March 7, 2016, I was aware the

CIA had a history of using undercover agents. I'd read MKUltra's Wikipedia page and parts of other writing on it, but not entire books or government documents. Months later, when, over eight months, I researched MKUltra for this book, I discovered a CIA–LSD–suicide–homicide thread that supported McKenna's argument that psychedelics are illegal not because the government wants to protect us from us but because they catalyze intellectual dissent.

On December 22, 1974, the *New York Times* reported that the CIA had conducted "a massive, illegal domestic intelligence operation during the Nixon Administration against the antiwar movement and other dissent groups." The government created two committees and a commission to investigate. And so, in the summer of 1975, people learned of Project MKUltra, which had existed under various names from 1950 to 1972, involved more than thirty institutions, and included tests in which, to research "behavior modification," LSD and other drugs were used on unwitting non-volunteers in a manner targeting "all social levels, high and low, native Americans and foreign"—or, by design, everyone—with no medical screening, follow-up, or even record-keeping. In spring 1977, more information became public, revealing that actually at least eighty institutions, including forty-four universities and twelve hospitals/clinics, had been involved. In Subproject 3, one of 149 subprojects, the CIA paid George H. White, who worked for the Anslinger-headed FBN, $40,000 a year to test LSD on random civilians. White set up "safe houses," as the CIA called them, in Greenwich Village, where he secretly dosed people with LSD, and in San Francisco, where he paid prostitutes to secretly dose customers with LSD while he watched via two-way mirror.

"Other experiments were equally offensive," said Senator Edward M. Kennedy in his opening remarks to the Senate hearing on MKUltra on August 3, 1977. "For example, heroin addicts were enticed into participating in LSD experiments in order to get a reward—heroin." Kennedy said, however, that "perhaps most disturbing of all was the fact that the extent of experimentation on human subjects was unknown. The records of all these activities were destroyed in January 1973, at the instruction of then CIA director Richard Helms." Kennedy, admirably, if futilely, stressed that, still: "The best safeguard against abuses in the future is a complete public account of the abuses of the past."

LSD testing on unwitting non-volunteers had not, I learned, been limited to the CIA. Appendix A of the public transcript of the three-hour five-minute hearing, at which only men spoke, was a novella-length report by the Senate Select Committee on Intelligence Activities titled "Testing and Use of Chemical and Biological Agents by the Intelligence Community." The report described eight classified projects, including two by the Army. In Project Derby Hat, the Army interrogated seven people in the Far East on LSD, including, in 1962, a "suspected Asian espionage agent" who received 6 micrograms per kilogram (or, if he weighed 140 pounds, around 2.5 tabs) of LSD one morning at 10:35 A.M., was "assisted to the interrogation table," according to the Army's "trip report"—a term used four times in the report, the first time in quotation marks—at 12:20 P.M., and interrogated until 3:30 A.M.

Like the hearing itself—in which seven current and former CIA employees were questioned, including Stansfield Turner, who said, "Let me emphasize that the MKULTRA events are twelve to twenty-five years in the past," and had been head of the CIA for only five months and was separated from Richard Helms by three heads—I found the Senate report darkly comical.

The two sentences in the report that eventually most attracted my attention were from a quote of a "lengthy staff study" published by the Army in 1959. The study analyzed data from LSD tests on more than a thousand Army soldiers since 1955 and concluded, quoted the Senate report:

> There has not been a single case of residual ill effect. Study of the prolific scientific literature on LSD-25 and personal communication between US Army Chemical Corps personnel and other researchers in this field have failed to disclose an authenticated instance of irreversible change being produced in normal humans by the drug.

This impressive finding on the safety of LSD, expressed in an internal Army text, has been supported by my personal experience as an emotionally unstable person with various mental problems who has enjoyed LSD at least eighty times since 2010 at measured doses of 20, 25, 37.5, 40, 50, 70, 87.5, 100, and 150 micrograms—and some higher, unmeasured doses—with only, I feel, positive, sanity-promoting effects. But in 1977, LSD had been a Schedule I drug for seven years. The Senate report commented on this disagreement between the Army and the government by arguing that the Army's conclusion had been based on incomplete data, because in 1959 they'd been unaware of "the circumstances surrounding Dr. Olson's death"—that Army scientist Frank Olson's 1953 death had been caused "at least in part," said the report, by LSD.

On day 6, we again heard no cases. In the waiting room, we napped and did things on our phones and computers, which we were encouraged to bring. We learned the other jury selected on day 1 was in a courtroom one room from our waiting room, which they sometimes entered to use our microwave. We theorized prosecutors had determined that, with our decreased indictment rate, it had become smarter—if the goal was to efficiently elicit indictments—to try the other jury first.

In a section titled "The Death of Dr. Frank Olson," the Senate report then examined what it called "the most tragic result of the testing of LSD by the CIA." On November 19, 1953, at a cabin in rural Maryland for a semi-annual "review and analysis conference," Frank Olson unwittingly ingested 70 micrograms of LSD, which CIA employee Robert Lashbrook had put into a bottle of liquor. Of the ten people there—seven Army, three CIA—all but two, from the Army, were dosed. Around twenty minutes later, Sidney Gottlieb, head of MKUltra, informed the group they'd ingested LSD. The report quoted Gottlieb saying they became "boisterous and laughing" and "could not continue the meeting or engage in sensible conversation." The report said, "Shortly after this experiment, Olson exhibited symptoms of paranoia and schizophrenia." After multiple meetings with a doctor in New York City with LSD experience and CIA clearance, "it was agreed that Olson should be placed under regular psychiatric care at an institution closer to his home" in Maryland. The next night, eight days after being dosed, Olson was in a tenth-floor room in Hotel Statler, across the street from Penn Station, with Lashbrook; at around 2:30 A.M., he "crashed through the closed window blind and the closed window," according to Lashbrook, who told police he didn't know why Olson committed suicide.

In the 1950s and 1960s, the CIA explained that Olson, who specialized in the use of microorganisms in biological warfare, had killed himself for unknown reasons. After the world learned, briefly in 1975 via the Rockefeller Commission and in more depth in the 1977 hearing and its appended report, that LSD had been involved, Olson's case was frequently, through the 1980s and 1990s, cited as an instance in which LSD led to psychosis and suicide, even in books reporting on the hellish details of MKUltra that the commission and hearing didn't mention—like *In the Sleep Room: The Story of the CIA Brainwashing Experiments in Canada* (1988), which described people being put into "chemical sleep" for weeks, hearing the same statements up to five hundred thousand times from football helmets or speakered pillows in what was called "automated psychotherapy," receiving unwitting injections of LSD, and undergoing amnesia-causing, electroshock-based "depatterning." *In the Sleep Room* referred to Frank Olson twice, saying on page 29 that he'd "been slipped a dose of LSD" and "had freaked out and jumped from the tenth-floor window of a New York hotel several days later" and on page 214 calling him "the army scientist who died of a fall from a hotel window shortly after being dosed with LSD."

As the world, for decades, associated LSD with insanity-caused suicide via the Frank Olson case, the 1977 Senate report's quote of the 1959 Army study deeming LSD safe remained obscure, unpublicized, and seemingly almost totally forgotten. A Google search, on March 21, 2017, of "There has not been a single case of residual ill effect" returned forty results, and all were reproductions of the entire MKUltra hearing itself except for a paper—"Cluster Headache, Dreaming & Neurogenesis"—self-published in 2006 by Peter May, meaning the quote has been reproduced by a Googlable source of newspaper, magazine, journal, book, blog, or other media only one time in forty years. May's paper, which argued for the use of psilocybin and other psychedelics to treat cluster headaches, included the Army quote with summaries of other studies that had found psychedelics to be relatively safe.

Researching Peter May, I found an article published by *Nature Medicine* in 2006 that quoted him saying cluster headaches felt "like someone is trying to pull your eye out." The article called them "suicide headaches" and said many sufferers had found "illegal drugs are their only choice," like May and, I knew, my friend Gian, who has ordered 5-MeO-DALT—a 42-atom compound created by Alexander Shulgin in 2004 that, being an analog of a Schedule I or II drug, can itself, under the Federal Analogue Act of 1986, be illegal—from the Czech Republic since 2015 to treat his cluster headaches. Unlike Gian, Peter May had no experience with psychedelics when, in 2002, after six months of research, he tried them for his cluster headaches—which he'd had since 1999—and experienced immediate success, reported the *Nature Medicine* article, which said the condition affected around one in one thousand people, making it, based on the Army study, more common than LSD causing "residual ill effect" when used wittingly.

Researching Frank Olson, I learned that, in 1994, evidence began to emerge that he didn't kill himself, though LSD may still have led to his death by inspiring him to speak out against an atrocity. That year, Eric Olson, who was nine when his dad died, had Frank Olson's body exhumed and a second autopsy ordered. James Starrs, who led the autopsy, concluded the body was "rankly and starkly suggestive of homicide," a finding absolving LSD from the death and so refuting the Senate report's only argument for why the Army study had been wrong. In 2001, then, the *New York Times Magazine* published an article reporting that Frank Olson's wife, Alice, remembered him, in the days after being dosed, being "in the grip of an ethical dilemma" and "withdrawn but not remotely psychotic" and that months earlier Olson may have confided to a psychiatrist that he'd witnessed something terrible, possibly a terminal experiment. I learned from the article that in 1997 the CIA "inadvertently declassified" an assassin's manual from the 1950s and that, from it, Eric Olson learned what the CIA seemed to have done to his dad—"dropped" him.

On day 7, we again heard no cases. During a long lunch break, I talked to Juror 12 on a bench outside Columbus Park. We recognized each other as he approached and he, a man in his sixties, sat. He was a playwright and had voted to dismiss around half the charges. I told him I was glad I hadn't entered the courtroom ahead of everyone and sat in one of the three elevated seats that faced the other twenty jurors and unwittingly become a secretary, foreperson, or assistant foreperson. We discussed Juror 8—who always voted to indict and never to deliberate and who seemed impatient when jurors asked questions—then he had a phone call from his daughter, who was meeting him nearby. After he left, I watched a squirrel unbury, unshell, and eat a peanut. That night, I noted that I was enjoying "suspecting both jurors who have talked to me to be working undercover for the CIA."

"Psychedelics are illegal *not* because a loving government is concerned that you may jump out of a third-story window," said McKenna in "Nature Is the Center of the Mandala" (1987). "Psychedelics are illegal because they dissolve opinion structures and culturally laid down models of behavior and information processing. They open you up to the possibility that everything you know is wrong." This was the reason he stressed most—and which can be viewed as underlying the other reasons discussed in this chapter—for why psychedelics are illegal. Because they're "catalysts of intellectual dissent." They make people question their behavior, other people's behaviors, and why things are how they are, and they do this while putting one in a state of mind open to change, novelty, and historical revisionism. This makes it difficult, observed McKenna, for societies—even democratic and especially dominator ones—to accept them, much less praise them, and we happen to live in a global dominator society.

McKenna got the terms "partnership" and "dominator" from Riane Eisler, who in *The Chalice and the Blade* (1987) proposed that beneath the "surface diversity of human culture" are two models of society—not communist/capitalist, matriarchal/patriarchal, religious/secular, or aboriginal/modern, but partnership/dominator. In the dominator model, one gender is ranked over the other in a bias that influences all relationships because it involves "the most fundamental difference in our species." In the partnership model, diversity, beginning with gender, isn't equated with inferiority or superiority; instead of ranking, there's "linking." Eisler's terms were deliberately gender-holistic—all humans can, and do, embody dominator values. The problem, she felt, was "not men as a sex" but the dominator model, in which "the Blade is idealized." In *The Chalice and the Blade*, which she observed was unlike most studies of society because it considered all of human history, Eisler argued that the dominator model began only around 7,000 years ago.

On day 8, we heard one case and saw, in an undercover video, our first accused person—a black man selling cocaine to an undercover Hispanic officer in a Dunkin' Donuts. I recorded most of this case as a Voice Memo. "So, if we're ready to vote on the one charge, please raise your hand; okay, that's everyone," said our

foreperson. The simplicity of our cases—officers buying or finding drugs—was not conducive to deliberation; in the fifteen to
twenty cases we heard, we deliberated three or four times, briefly,
with two to five people speaking, then stopped getting enough
votes to deliberate. "So then on the charge of the criminal sale
of a substance in the third degree, if you want to vote to indict,
please raise your hand." With twenty jurors looking at her, she
counted the votes. "Okay, that's fifteen." Juror 1, our secretary,
wrote the voting result on paper, then left to tell the judge we'd
finished voting. The judge entered and said, "All right, folks,
we're going to break for lunch until two thirty."

At least 35,000 years ago, humans in Eurasia began to carve
female figurines from bone, stone, and ivory. The oldest known
example, the Venus of Hohle Fels, was found in Germany in
2009. Instead of a head, the fig-size, 35,000- to 40,000-year-old
mammoth-tusk sculpture had a polished ring, probably indicating it had been suspended as a pendant. Archaeologist Marija
Gimbutas (1921–1994) estimated in her posthumous book *The
Living Goddesses* (1999) that around three thousand female and
genderlessly zoomorphic figurines had been found in the Upper
Paleolithic, from 40,000 to 12,000 years ago, a period with no
male figurines. Popular culture and most books and textbooks
explain that they're either, Eisler wrote, "an ancient analogue for
today's *Playboy* magazine" or "expressions of a primitive fertility
cult."

An example of the sex object interpretation is in "She's Still
a Pin-up after 35,000 Years," an article on NBCNews.com that
quoted archaeologist Paul Mellars, whose commentary on the
sculpture was published in the issue of *Nature* announcing
the discovery: "Paleolithic *Playboy*? We just don't know how it

was used at this point, but the object's size meant it fit well in someone's hand." The pornography interpretation also occurs in *Cave of Forgotten Dreams* (2010) by Werner Herzog, who brought 3-D cameras into Chauvet Cave in France to film 30,000- to 32,000-year-old art. For insight into the cave's only human representation—a bison-zoomorphized drawing of thighs and vulva—the documentary cut to the director of the cave's research project, who showed a copy of a 27,000- to 30,000-year-old limestone figurine (with a characteristic hexagram of bulges around a pregnant belly) and said its bottom half resembled the drawing. Then his voice was muted and Herzog voice-over narrated, "There seems to have existed a visual convention extending all the way beyond *Baywatch*." In 2010, I had not consciously heard of or suspected the existence of an ancient religion with a female God, so, though Herzog's interpretation seemed unconvincing, I lacked a better explanation. I remember telling myself maybe the figurines really were sex objects.

Four years later, when I researched this topic for Tao Of Terence—for a post in which I encouraged people to "get stoned and read *The Chalice and the Blade*"—I began to realize that people with busy, public, meaningful lives (embedded with families and tribes in densely symbiotic ecosystems, tending and harvesting and hunting and preparing food, monitoring the stars and seasons and other life-forms) probably wouldn't spend hours carving a tiny pendant to help them masturbate. Gimbutas, who wrote four books on the Goddess, observed that due to "modern cultural programming," people associated "nakedness" with "sexual enticement" but that the female body symbolized many other functions, including "the procreative, nurturing, and life enhancing."

As I read books by Eisler, Gimbutas, and others, I became convinced, as those authors argued, that the figurines symbolized the universe's life-giving force by emphasizing the female body's unique parts and abilities—and that, with other evidence, they suggested the existence of a widespread, cross-cultural, female-deitied religion that began in the Upper Paleolithic or earlier. One reason humans worshipped a female deity was probably, I learned, because only women give birth. Prehistoric humans, noticing that life emerged only from women—who alone nursed that life—naturally developed a worldview featuring this fact. In *When God Was a Woman* (1976), sculptress Merlin Stone (1931–2011) shared another reason why people, for tens of thousands of years, seemed to have worshipped female deities; citing studies of aboriginals by James Frazer, Jacquetta Hawkes, and others, Stone wrote that "as the earliest concepts of religion developed, they probably took the form of ancestor worship," which meant mother worship because people had not connected sex and babies so did not know they had fathers.

After agriculture developed from 12,000 to 10,000 years ago in the Fertile Crescent, people there and beyond, from England to Pakistan, continued for at least three millennia, I learned, to create female figurines, though they now lived not nomadically but, as at Jericho, in stone-foundationed, mud-brick houses with thousands of others. It was during this Neolithic period, when gender equality was "the general norm," wrote Eisler, that most of the technologies of civilization—farming, stockbreeding, pottery, ceramics, megalithic architecture, metallurgy, wheeled vehicles, textiles, writing—developed. Eisler, who was born in 1937 in Austria and fled the Nazi takeover of her country when she was a child, going to Cuba then the States, called this "one of the best kept historical secrets"—that advancement doesn't require war.

In *Earliest Civilizations of the Near East* (1965), James Mellaart (1925–2012) identified Çatalhöyük, where people lived from 9,400 to 7,500 years ago, as the most advanced culture and largest settlement, with up to eight thousand residents, of this period. From 1961 to 1963, Mellaart excavated an acre of the 33.5-acre main mound of the double mound of Çatalhöyük. He found matrilineal and matrilocal organization—the woman's platform for sitting, working, and sleeping was always on the east side of the house, whereas the man's shifted and was smaller—and that, based on stone-and-clay figurines, wall paintings, and other art, the city's "principal deity" was "a goddess who is shown in her three aspects, as a young woman, a mother giving birth or as an old woman." People probably had gained the concept of father—a stone plaque showed a couple embracing on the left and a child-holding woman on the right—and now also made male figurines (Mellaart found thirty-three female, eight male), but Goddess worship seemed to remain the most important practice. At least 40 of 139 buildings excavated were, in Mellaart's view, shrines, including one with wall drawings of women birthing, which Gimbutas called "probably one of the most sacrosanct events in Neolithic religion," and the rest were homes. Shrines, homes, and middens formed one accreting, doorless, streetless, leaderless, egalitarian city enterable only by ladder from each building's different-elevationed roof.

The commonest motif in Çatalhöyükian art was the male cow, or bull, which Mellaart interpreted in 1967 to represent "male power." Gimbutas stressed throughout her work that, in the pre-dominator cultures of Anatolia and Europe, the bull was a Goddess symbol, conveying becoming and regeneration, because of the resemblance of its head-and-horns, or bucranium, to the uterus and fallopian tubes. McKenna in *Food of the Gods* argued the cow and bull symbolized both the Goddess and the mushroom because Çatalhöyükians recognized the mushroom as "the physical connection" to the Goddess and, since it sprouted from cow dung, viewed it, like milk, as a product of cattle. Abandoned

around 7,500 years ago for unknown reasons, with people possibly relocating to the island of Crete, maybe because they sensed
the violence to come on the mainland, Çatalhöyük was the last
civilization, theorized McKenna, that was continuously informed
by "the gnosis of the boundary-dissolving plant hallucinogens."

On day 9, a Friday, Juror 11 said bye to me because, she said, she
wouldn't be there Monday, the last day. This made sense, I felt, if
she worked for the CIA; her expensive time was subject to repri-
oritization. Maybe she or her boss had determined I was closed
off to a certain degree in terms of talkativeness—as I was during
this time, being focused on my book—making me not a good
investment in befriending, and then it took three days of paperwork to move her off the project. We heard no cases that day.

The dominator model, which previously existed in balanced and
controlled form, emerged in a sustained, whole-society, assailing
manner around 7,000 years ago, argued Eisler and Gimbutas
and others. At this time, various groups of dominator-style people from the north, including the Kurgans in Europe, Luwians in
Anatolia, and Hittites in the Fertile Crescent—called, as a group,
Indo-Europeans—began to invade the Goddess-worshipping
civilizations in the south, first in the Near East, then in Anatolia,
and, spreading west over millennia, throughout Europe. They
worshipped male deities, rode horses and war chariots, were
hierarchic, patrilineal, patrilocal, and pastoral, and had lighter
skin and were bigger than those in the south. They associated
black with death, unlike the preexisting people in Europe and
Anatolia—Old Europeans—who viewed black, wrote Gimbutas
in *The Language of the Goddess* (1989), as "the color of fertility, the

color of damp caves and rich soil, of the womb of the Goddess where life begins."

In the Sumerian and Egyptian civilizations, which began 6,000 to 5,000 years ago and, wrote Eisler, "are celebrated in our high school and college textbooks as marking the beginnings of Western civilization," people still worshipped female deities, but male deities began to dominate. Around the Eighteenth Dynasty, 3,570 years ago, when Egyptian women were no longer part of the religious clergy, some people in the Near East—where a supreme deity, known by many names, had already, for millennia, been "revered as Goddess—much as people think of God," wrote Stone—began to worship a male deity named Yahweh, who, according to the Bible, told his laws to Moses, who wrote them down and gave them to the Levites, a Hebrew tribe. "Perhaps the most shocking laws of all were those that declared that a woman was to be stoned or burned to death for losing her virginity before marriage, a factor never mentioned in other law codes of the Near East," wrote Stone, who observed that the Bible "purposely glossed over" the Goddess's gender, calling her Elohim—"in the masculine gender, to be translated as god"—but that the Koran, the bible of Islam, did not: "Allah will not tolerate idolatry . . . the pagans pray to females."

The Levites, tyrannically leading the other eleven Hebrew tribes, invaded Canaan—an area around the size and mirror-reversed shape of California—and instated their laws over the survivors of their rampage. "So Joshua massacred the population of the whole region—the hill country, the Negeb, the Shepelah, the watersheds," according to the Bible. The laws targeted Goddess worship because in Goddess-worshipping societies, daughters inherited name, title, and property—and because, even though the concept of father had been known for millennia, women called *qadishtu*—"holy women"—continued to birth fatherless babies by living in temple-complexes where, coming and going as they desired, they had sex with various men. This was "probably the underlying reason for the resentment of the worship of the Goddess," wrote Stone, who stressed that the sexism of the laws was political, not religious, having nothing to do with the mystery of life.

After the initial invasions from 7,000 to 4,800 years ago, the Goddess religion survived, in places, as the popular religion for millennia; it was not until the Levites and then the rise of Christianity that it was, in the first century, "finally suppressed and nearly forgotten." For the next two millennia, Yahweh-based, anti-partnership ideas continued to spread in the form of the Crusades, the Inquisition, witch hunts, all-male clergies, and, among other memes, the Adam and Eve myth—in which Yahweh absurdly punished women with pain in childbirth and to be ruled by men. Around 350 years ago, the United States was founded "under God" and around 100 years ago, American women gained the right to vote. On November 8, 2016, at 7:30 P.M., the *New York Times* estimated Hillary Clinton had a more than 80 percent chance of becoming the president. By midnight, it was under 5 percent. The next morning, Donald Trump, embodying the dominator model arguably more than any previous candidate, was, in the lowest voter turnout since 1996, elected the forty-fifth consecutive male president of the United States, which, out of 196 countries and 5,000 aboriginal groups, had by far the largest military budget—triple the second-place country, China, which had four times the population.

Knowing this narrative, the past 4,800 years can be viewed as an inconsistent, unpredictable, many-threaded, unguaranteed but achievable recovery—instead of a hopeless continuation of a seemingly always cruel and violent human history, like I mostly suspected before learning all this—from the overexpression of the dominator model, which for 7,000 years has been erasing evidence and memory, across civilizations and continents, of the Goddess religion and its partnership way of life.

We also heard no cases on day 10, when I brought my computer for the first time. The other days, I'd hand-edited pages of this book and read others' books. On days 3 and 4, I'd read *LSD: My Problem Child* (1980) by Albert Hofmann, who was born in 1906, created LSD from a compound (lysergic acid) made by ergot (fungi from the genus *Claviceps*) in 1938, answered "What general medical uses might LSD be marketed for in the future?" with "Very small doses, perhaps 25 micrograms, could be useful as a euphoriant or antidepressant" in 1976, and died in 2008. I'd used 0.3 grams of baked cannabis every day except day 8, when I used half an old, degraded tab of LSD—maybe around 40 micrograms—and day 10, when, on my way to Chinatown, at 9:53 A.M., I used the other half. On this dose, I felt more outgoing and curious, and less inflamed, than normal. Walking around on my lunch break, I enjoyed "remarkable mobility," I typed in notes .rtf at 2:08 P.M., in my hips and legs. "Still feel lucid," I typed at 4:56 P.M. in my room, where I worked on this book's psilocybin chapter, researched inflammation, and, at 10:32 P.M., slept.

Besides cannabis, we'd heard only two cases with psychedelics—psilocybin and LSD. Both cases also involved heroin and/or cocaine and, unsurprisingly, we indicted all four drugs without deliberation. Cannabis, which can be almost as powerful as psilocybin and LSD when eaten, had been involved in almost every case. I was reminded of this prevalence when I read "Legalize It All," which was published a month after jury duty; the report, subtitled "How to Win the War on Drugs," quoted the director of the ACLU from 1978 to 2001 as saying that "the drug war couldn't be sustained" if cannabis was legal because the "vanishingly small" use of other drugs couldn't justify police and prison spending. Researching prison, I learned two countries had more than a million prisoners in 2015, the United States with 2.15 million and China with 1.65 million.

It's unknown how the dominator model became so out-of-control. Maybe the human species is so precariously balanced that a combination of seemingly small factors, like horse domestication, invoking military advantage and the desire to ride and be nomadic, tipped entire societies into dominator mode. And as societies abandoned the cross-gender reverence of women to worship the larger-so-better-at-war gender, things deteriorated further and the partnership model was forgotten. In *Food of the Gods*, McKenna argued that the equilibrium was maintained by psychedelics and their connection to "the archetype of the Goddess and hence to the partnership style."

One of the last places in Western society where psychedelics were regularly, if seldomly, used was Eleusis, where the most famous Mystery was practiced. In the Greco-Roman world, a Mystery was a religion in which "the individual was afforded an experience of personal communion with deity," wrote Carl Ruck in *Sacred Mushrooms of the Goddess* (2006). The Eleusinian Mystery is theorized to have been practiced openly for millennia on Crete by the Minoans, a partnership civilization, or gylany, which may have been seeded from Çatalhöyük, before it began to be practiced semi-secretly on the mainland around 3,500 years ago—fifty years after Abraham, six hundred miles away, began promoting Yahweh, according to an estimate from *When God Was a Woman*. For 1,900 years, people in Athens who spoke Greek and had not killed anyone outside of war had the option to experience the Eleusinian Mysteries, whose Goddesses were Demeter and Persephone. Completing the Lesser Mystery in February allowed one to be an initiate, nineteen months later, in the Greater Mystery, which occurred over nine days in September, including a day walking fourteen miles from Athens to Eleusis and a night stoned on a drink called *kykeon* in a building called the *telestêrion* that, after multiple reconstructions, held thousands and which contained a small chamber that one initiate entered at a time.

Alaric the Visigoth destroyed the *telestêrion* in 396 AD, four years after a Christian Roman emperor deemed Christianity the official religion and closed the Eleusinian Mystery. Before the experience became illegal, Pythagoras, Sophocles, Plato, Aristotle, Cicero, and others went, drank *kykeon*, and published positive, awed thoughts on their trips. In *The Road to Eleusis* (1978), Wasson, Hofmann, and Ruck theorized *kykeon* contained an LSD-like compound made by ergot, which grows on rye, barley, and other grasses. Wasson quoted Aristides the Rhetor, calling the experience "new, astonishing, inaccessible to rational cognition."

In May, when I was working on this book's DMT chapter, I encountered a juror who I'd also seen in public in March, the night after jury duty ended, when, walking in opposite directions, we'd waved. He was the juror who, on day 1, asked why we were indicting a dinky knife. This time we stopped to talk.

He said he forgot to tell me something last time. We'd been the only two, he said, who voted to dismiss on every charge. As prologue, it seemed, to explaining why he'd voted to dismiss all, he said he'd "studied law and philosophy" and trailed off, looking at me. He asked how I felt about the experience. I said good, pro-

ductive. As officers learned juries were dismissing cannabis felonies, they would become reluctant to try to prosecute them—to
make the arrest, do the paperwork, go to Chinatown, sit on a
witness stand—and as people in the cannabis trade learned
juries weren't indicting cannabis felonies, they'd become bolder
in their investments and marketing, and eventually cannabis,
barring being targeted by a billion- or trillion-dollar industry or
organization, could become legal again; with cannabis, the entry
psychedelic, legal, the others could follow. My votes supported
this trend, so I felt productive.

We were in Washington Square Park. We discussed how,
in the back row, he'd seen every vote. He said most jurors had
seemed to try to vote with the majority and that gradually more
had voted to dismiss cannabis charges. He was the only juror I'd
encountered since jury duty ended; he seemed to want to talk a
little more but didn't, and we said bye.

CANNABIS

1

On February 14, 2016, I learned from Tracy that Botanical Dimensions, the nonprofit founded in 1985 by Kathleen Harrison and Terence McKenna to "collect, protect, propagate and understand plants of ethno-medical significance," had opened a library in Northern California. Four months and four days had passed since I smoked Tracy's DMT, and in three days I would begin writing this book. Investigating Botanical Dimensions's website, I noticed the organization's curvy logo—made of eight pairs of curly parts connected by a squarish ring into an asymmetrical, wreathlike design, like a vine-inflected yin-yang—and that Harrison was co-teaching a plant-drawing class at the library on July 2, my thirty-third birthday.

2

In "Who Is Cannabis?" (2015), Kathleen Harrison observed that humans are skilled at consciously and unconsciously noticing qualities about other humans and suggested we use our "groking" abilities on other species too, instead of thinking, "Oh, more green stuff that's really hard to tell apart from all the other green stuff." From her twenty-five-minute talk, I learned:

- Harrison, who was sixty-seven, had "never left her love of cannabis." When she wanted to "climb onto her magic carpet" and go above the situation to reflect on and write about it, she smoked cannabis.

- It surprised her how many people she met who said cannabis made them paranoid. "I think it's become a meme, you know—'It makes me paranoid.'"

- In terms of staying well in a "seemingly crazy modern world," she most appreciated cannabis for the "comfort" and "solace" it provided.

- She was not social with cannabis; for her, it was "a meditative herb."

- She always greeted cannabis as her "big sister." Her impulse was to rest against cannabis's shoulder and say, "Ah, thank you, you're here too, that reminds me that the world is not on my shoulders, it's on *our* shoulders, there are bigger entities than me trying to do the little part to save it every day."

- People she'd spent time with in Latin America appealed daily, she'd noticed, in prayers and songs, to Santa María, a deity viewed by some practitioners of the ayahuasca-based religion Santo Daime as accessible through cannabis: "To be soothed, because life is hard. To remember the beauty so they can do the next hard thing."

- In Harrison's view, cannabis's millennia-long relationship with humans showed it wanted to be with us. Cannabis had offered herself as fiber, food, medicine, and "medicine for the spirit," helping us "balance out all the alienation and mechanization and institutional-enforced suffering."

3

Terence McKenna encountered cannabis in 1965, when he was eighteen. He'd inherited "the programming" from his "middle-class straight parents" that "the road to hell was paved" with it, but he'd also read Burroughs, Ginsberg, and others with different opinions. As an adolescent, he'd been "what they call 'a nervous child'"; now he realized that smoking "a small amount of vegetable material" could make him "a reasonably functioning member of the community." Within months, cannabis became "the central practice" of his life. "And it has remained so up until just two or three months ago when, under the pressure of my apparently dissolving marriage, I stopped smoking in order to see, really, what sort of effect it would have," he said in "Cannabis Trialogue" (1991). He explained that he and Kathleen had been in couples therapy with someone "who seemed to be a very skilled psychotherapist" but had "no sophistication whatsoever about cannabis." This conversation would happen:

PSYCHOTHERAPIST: Well, now, how many times a day do you do this?

MCKENNA: Eh, ten to fourteen.

PSYCHOTHERAPIST: And how many years have you been doing this?

MCKENNA: Well, twenty-five, twenty-six, twenty-seven?

Cannabis was impeding the therapeutic process due to its effects on his therapist's attitude toward him, so he stopped smoking it. "And I'm happy to report that, though I was at that time the heaviest and most continuous cannabis user that I have ever known or ever heard of, it was no big deal. I simply stopped smoking it, and took up reading in the evenings, and it seemed to have no impact on my psychological organization at all except that, I must say, my dream life became considerably more interesting."

4

In his book's preface, Chris Duvall said he wrote *Cannabis* to try to understand how cannabis "gained its cosmopolitan status," growing on "all inhabited landmasses to about 60 degrees latitude, a distribution broader than any other crop." In "Ancient *Cannabis*," his book's second chapter, he observed that cannabis evolved tens of millions of years before humans.

5

On March 1, sixteen days after learning of Botanical Dimensions's library and the plant-drawing class, I began serving ten days of jury duty, which I examined in the previous chapter. I was surprised so many jurors voted to dismiss cannabis felonies, but also unsurprised, because I knew humans had enjoyed cannabis for millennia and that, in the United States, after almost a century of criminalization, it was quickly becoming relegalized, with Washington and Colorado unbanning it in 2012, Alaska and Oregon and Washington, D.C., in 2014, and other states expected to follow.

6

Around 50 million years ago, when our ancestors resembled long-limbed squirrels, India began colliding into south-central Asia, where proto-cannabis lived, creating the Himalayas over tens of millions of years, during which, elsewhere on the planet, monkeys and then apes evolved. The impact moved some proto-cannabis populations closer, through changes in elevation and latitude, to the sun. These populations evolved more THC, a 53-atom compound acting in part as "sunscreen," wrote Duvall, against ultraviolet-B radiation. India finished colliding into Asia around eleven million years ago. By six million years ago, when proto-humans had begun walking upright but still lived in trees, cannabis had evolved into a genus of two species, indica and sativa, producing versatile fiber, nutritious seeds, and resin, flowers, leaves, stems, and roots with at least 554 different compounds, of which 113 were cannabinoids, including, most abundantly, psychoactive THC and anti-inflammatory CBD.

7

In 2015, a paper in *Emotion* observed that clinical depression and anxiety are "associated with higher levels of proinflammatory cytokines." The paper shared the results of a study at Berkeley in which 105 undergraduates answered questionnaires online and later had their IL-6 (a pro-inflammatory cytokine) levels measured. One questionnaire measured "positive emotions in their daily lives." Of those measured—amusement, awe, compassion, contentment, joy, love, pride—awe, surprisingly, had "the strongest relationship" with IL-6 levels, followed, not closely, by joy, pride, and contentment. The paper said there was probably a "bidirectional relationship between positive affect and cytokine production," or, in other words, probably (1) decreasing inflam-

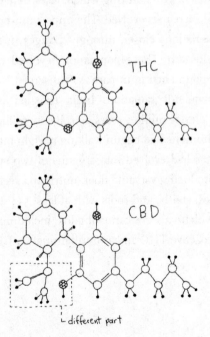

THC

CBD

└ different part

mation via diet and environment and exercise increases one's capacity to feel awe and other positive emotions and (2) positive emotions, especially awe, decrease inflammation. Awe, I learned after some research, was measured by numerical ratings of these sentences:

I often feel awe.

I see beauty all around me.

I feel wonder almost every day.

I often look for patterns in the objects around me.

I have many opportunities to see the beauty of nature.

I seek out experiences that challenge my understanding of
the world.

Reading those sentences, I thought of how I never felt awe, and almost never felt wonder, before incorporating psychedelics and McKenna's ideas into my life. I thought of how I saw beauty all around me but mostly only in advertisements—a kind of "beauty" determined by corporations that made me feel exploited, exploitative, inadequate, and alienated. I thought of how I did not especially seek experiences to challenge my worldview, rarely went to see the beauty of nature, and left New York City only for book-related events or to visit my parents in Taipei, another dense metropolis.

8

On April 22, a month and eight days after my jury duty ended, I bought a ticket for the plant-drawing class—"Botanical Illustration: Learning to Really See Plants & Draw Them"—and on May 2, embedded in notes.rtf, I started a plant-drawing diary. Eight days later, I began drafting this chapter, on cannabis. Unsure what form to use, but knowing I wanted a change from the previous chapters, I contemplated and waited and experimented, organizing and disassembling and recombining information. Over thirteen months and four drafts, adapting to feedback from my editor, a thirty-three-part fractal structure formed with ten of the parts—1, 5, 8, 15, 18, 21, 23, 26, 32, 33—telling a story set from February, when I began writing this book, to July, when I flew to California to visit Kathleen Harrison.

9

From six to three million years ago, our ancestors began to spend less time in trees and evolved into the *Homo*, or human, genus. From three million to around 300,000 years ago, the human brain-size tripled; in *Food of the Gods*, McKenna quoted biologists Charles Lumsden and Edward Wilson, calling this "perhaps the fastest advance recorded for any complex organ in the whole history of life" and theorized psilocybin catalyzed the evolution. To the millions of humans who lived during these 27,000 centuries, when knowledge on how to live in optimized symbiosis with thousands of life-forms was passed down over more than 110,000 generations in an unbroken, unconscious process, like in salamanders, vultures, and other animals, the rapid change was probably impossible to notice.

10

In its "General Discussion" section, the *Emotion* paper said it contributed to "a growing body of work" showing that positive emotions "not only feel good, they are good for the body" and that awe was associated with "curiosity and a desire to explore." The 2015 paper referenced a 2006 paper in *The Journal of Positive Psychology* that said people "experience awe when confronted with a novel, highly complex stimulus that current knowledge structures cannot fully assimilate." The 2006 paper referenced a 2003 paper in *Cognition and Emotion* that said awe hadn't "been shown to have a distinctive facial expression" and that psychology "has had surprisingly little to say about awe." The psychedelic literature has had much to say, I've noticed, on awe. "Awe leads to humility," wrote Kathleen Harrison in a 2009 essay. "It gets you outside yourself, and puts your story in appropriate perspective as an instant in a very long saga, the one we're all in together. That we humans, and human cultures, are embedded in natural cycles becomes obvious. The question—and psychedelics certainly raise more questions than they answer—is how do we best 'wear' and 'articulate' that fact of being creatures with unusual agency in nature's timeless epic."

11

Homo sapiens, or anatomically modern humans, evolved at least 280,000 years ago in Africa. Multiple times in our first 206,000 years, groups of us left Africa in various directions, surviving for varying amounts of time and sometimes reproducing with other species in the *Homo* genus, like Neanderthals and Denisovans.

Around 74,000 years ago, Mount Toba in Sundaland—a landmass that existed where the Indonesian islands are now—ejected 670 cubic miles of material over nine to fourteen days in the largest explosive eruption in at least nineteen million years. Six years of "volcanic winter" that "could have decimated most modern human populations," wrote Stanley Ambrose in a 1998 paper in *Journal of Human Evolution*, was followed by a millennium of "the coldest, driest climate" of the past 500,000 to a million years. The human population fell from around one hundred thousand to probably between two and eight thousand. The traumatized survivors, who "would have found refuge in isolated tropical pockets, mainly in Equatorial Africa," wrote Ambrose, were our ancestors.

Around 72,000 years ago, estimated a 2016 paper in *Nature*, a group of us, again, left Africa, entering Eurasia. At some point—30,000 years ago, estimated Duvall—we encountered cannabis in the Himalayas. The next 20,000 years, as we drew on cave walls and sculpted female figurines and began living in permanent settlements, cannabis went where we went. Without planes or websites, cannabis took longer than *Salvia divinorum*, which also once existed in montane isolation, to become our international symbiont—millennia instead of years, reaching the Black Sea by 16,000 years ago; Yangmingshan, the mountains north of Taipei where pottery fragments have been found with "the imprint of a cord-like material thought to be of hemp," wrote Leslie Iversen in *The Science of Marijuana* (2008), by 12,000 years ago; Italy and Japan by 10,000 years ago.

12

Cannabinoids are compounds that interact with cannabinoid receptors, of which at least two types exist—CB1 mediates psychoactivity and CB2 mediates immune-system functions, like inflammation. Despite evolving long before cannabis—as early as 600 million years ago in sea squirts—these receptors are named after cannabis because compounds that interact with them were discovered in cannabis before, in 1992 with the discovery of the 62-atom compound anandamide, in animals.

In 2010, a paper in the *British Journal of Pharmacology* asked if other plants besides cannabis made phytocannabinoids. It answered yes—β-caryophyllene, a 39-atom compound, was in cannabis and many other plants and had "strong anti-inflammatory and analgesic effects in wild-type mice but not in CB2 receptor knockout mice"—but not THC. "The question remains as to why *Cannabis sativa* L. appears to be the only plant that produces a metabolite (Δ9-THC acid) that readily leads to its decarboxylation product Δ9-THC, which is the most potent phytocannabinoid activator of the CB1 receptor," concluded the paper.

One answer could be that other plants with THC remain undiscovered; around two thousand plant species are discovered annually, according to a 2016 paper in *Phytotaxa* that estimated around 374,000 plant species are known. Another answer could be that there are so many possible compounds that, even with so many species, some can still be expected to have unique compounds; or, in other words, that cannabis is a special plant and so, as we attracted it—because it thrives, wrote Duvall, "in recently disturbed, fertile soil"—it attracted us and when we found it we prized and grew it.

13

Between 12,000 and 10,000 years ago, some humans began farming and raising animals in an area between Europe, Asia, and Africa around the size of three Californias in "a pluralistic process with initial domestication of various crops and livestock occurring, sometimes multiple times in the same species, across the entire region," according to a 2011 paper on the origins of agriculture. Their descendants multiplied and spread and became "modern people" who comprise our global culture. Other humans continued living like they had for seemingly ever—in a timeless trance, outside history, like snails and leopards and other animals, hunting and foraging and gathering and doing limited, if any, farming. These people, without changing, became, in terms of this book, "aboriginal people." Aboriginals lacked the hierarchy-and-material-obsessed, nature-ignoring knowledge generated by millennia of dominator-style civilizations—a knowledge ranging from egregiously wrong to complicatedly confusing to stimulating and useful, like knowing down to atoms how life builds itself—and modern people increasingly lacked the knowledge gained from living in nature for millions of years, but many of them, like Kathleen Harrison, were learning and teaching it.

14

In late 2014, I learned from Weston A. Price, a modern person from Canada, that aboriginals who lived like their ancestors, outside agriculture and civilization, were, without toothbrushes or dentists, nearly free of tooth decay—a major problem for modern people—and that in aboriginals "practically all teeth form and erupt normally, including the third molars." I learned aboriginal children born to parents who'd switched to a modern diet suffered lowered fertility and mentation, deformed feet, and other types of cumulative degeneration, like underdeveloped bottom halves of heads, causing the long, thin faces and crowded mouths that, already, in the 1930s, characterized modern people. Like seemingly everyone, I'd accepted the absurd-seeming reality that humans have evolved through natural selection to grow debilitatingly impacted wisdom and other teeth requiring surgical removal. Now the absurdity resolved to instructive, extrapolatable clarity as I learned this was degenerative.

Since sedentizing into increasingly grain-based, pesticide-using, factory-farming, automobile-infested, plant-deprived, plasticized, sterilized, sunlight-less, virtual-reality-like civilizations, we have also, besides degenerating physically, become gradually more dysbiotic, diseased, malnourished, and inflamed. A 2007 paper in *Clinical & Experimental Immunology* called inflammation "part of the nonspecific immune response that occurs in reaction to any type of bodily injury." Inflamed, our bodies distract our minds with pain and discomfort instead of feeling like easily controllable, lightweight tools that we can put down when we want to explore the metaphysical part of existence. Inflammation encourages the development of bleak worldviews by sucking attention toward matter, making us feel less dimensional, like we are only our bodies and not our minds. As degeneration and inflammation worsened by the millennium, century, and decade, in increasingly steep curves, cannabis became more useful, helpful, powerful, and magical-seeming.

In "Art, Drugs & Consciousness" (2012), a discussion in Brooklyn, Hamilton Morris said he once tried a drug, invented for dieting purposes, that blocked his cannabinoid receptors. "You become miserable," he said. The drug, a 51-atom compound called rimonabant, worked for weight loss but failed overall because people became "suicidally depressed," among other problems. "You don't think you're high all the time," said Morris, "but in some sense you are." I imagine that, as twenty-first century, chronically inflamed degenerates, we are at least a little less high, on average, than 90,000, 15,000, 5,000, or 500 years ago—that we each have the opportunity to become gradually more stoned just by weaning ourselves off civilization, nature-ward.

15

On May 21, walking from Bobst Library to my apartment, I collected fourteen leaves. "I started drawing the most circular leaf, and it seemed more complex than I had unconsciously assumed," I typed in my plant-drawing diary that night. After looking at it for minutes, the leaf began to seem like a vaguely pulsing organism instead of a motionless shape. The next night, I learned the leaf had twenty-two and nineteen points on each side, with the bottommost point being both twenty-third and twentieth, and that eight and seven veins went left and right from its midrib. I was surprised by the complexity—that 22/19, 23/20, and 8/7 were irreducible and that each point protruded from a protrusion, like beaks from birds' heads, instead of just sticking out from the leaf like I'd obliviously assumed. I was surprised I could count, between the smallest veins, each tiny green shape that seemed two-dimensional and roundedly geometric, fitting amid one another like weathered blocks. I could keep looking, I knew, into the leaf, like in those YouTube videos that zoom into fractals for hours. Staring, with a microscope, at the same place, I'd keep discovering new details.

16

In *The Fractal Geometry of Nature* (1982), Benoit Mandelbrot (1924–2010) wrote that nature's patterns are "so irregular and fragmented" that, compared to standard geometry, the natural world was "an altogether different level of complexity"—referring to how stars and galaxies are not evenly distributed, hearts not spheres, mountains not cones, bark not smooth. "The nature of fractals is meant to be gradually discovered by the reader, not revealed in a flash by the author," wrote Mandelbrot, who invented the word "fractal" from a Latin adjective—*fractus*—whose corresponding verb—*frangere*—meant "to create irregular fragments."

Nature builds with fractal shapes and processes, which graph in jagged patterns that seem random but are to some degree predictable. Fractals are common in nature but, because humans have downloaded many non-fractal forms from the imagination into the universe, uncommon in culture. Things humans do not consciously influence remain fractal—weather, Brownian motion, spider webs, the wending paths of birds. The roughness of sidewalks at micrometer levels, where humans haven't smoothed the concrete, is fractal, but sidewalks are not. On Earth, only with humans have strangely non-fractal objects appeared—doors, cubicles, streets, straight-line-flying drones. But humans, being natural, are also fractal and so enjoy behaving and creating fractally. Bobst Library looks like a simple cube from far away, but up close one can see that it's vertically fissured like a tree trunk, though, with exact spacing and right angles, less fractal than a tree.

Fractal can be a point of view. Most things can be viewed as fractal. In terms of being self-similar at different scales—a characteristic of fractals—a refrigerator is fractal in that, as a plastic, hollow container, it contains objects similar to itself, like how an animal (organs in skin) contains cells (organelles in membranes). Zooming in more, though, into one of its containers, one encounters things that suddenly aren't refrigerator-like—

sauerkraut, miso—and now the refrigerator seems more obviously unnatural. Fractal, in this way, can be a subjective word. I sometimes use it as a synonym for "natural-seeming" when considering behaviors, systems, visual art, writing, and music. Chopin's music is rhythmically more fractal to me than what I've heard of Bach's, for example, because it often uses polyrhythms—sustained passages of four notes against three and three against two, instances of 7/6, 14/3, 22/12, and other oddities—while Bach's is often reducible to 2/1, an unnaturally simple temporal relationship between sounds.

Fractals are explorable. In a fractal object—a galaxy, a leaf—one can travel through scale in either direction, discovering new properties and patterns and life-forms. Zooming into a dot in the sky, one could discover a supercluster. Zooming into a dot in the supercluster, one would discover a galaxy. Zooming into one of the galaxy's billions of dots, one would be a little surprised to find not another enormous selection of dots but an intensely glowing sphere—or two or more in binary and multiple systems—orbited by a small number of tiny, dim spheres. Zooming into a sphere, one would be surprised to find not more dots or spheres following the laws of physics but, seemingly hidden there, in the meter scale of size, complicatedly shaped objects traveling in desultory, anti-gravitational ways. Zooming into an animal, one would find, at the micrometer level, more unpredictably moving, irregular shapes. In this way, planets, animals, and microorganisms are hidden far inside the fractal of the universe.

"Time is a fractal, or has a fractal structure," wrote McKenna in a 1991 essay. "All times, moments, months and millennia, have a pattern; the same pattern. This pattern is the structure within which, upon which, events 'undergo the formality of actually occurring,' as Whitehead used to say. The pattern recurs on every level. A love affair, the fall of an empire, the death agony of a protozoan, all occur within the context of this always the same but ever different pattern. All events are resonances of other events, in other parts of time, and at other scales of time."

If time is a fractal, the human genus is hidden inside ten million years, *Homo sapiens* inside a million years, individual humans inside millennia and centuries, thoughts inside seconds and minutes, and feelings, both briefer and longer lasting than thoughts, inside deciseconds, seconds, minutes, hours, days, weeks, months, seasons, years, and decades.

17

In China, a millennium before Jesus, a group of people went as deep into their study of time, McKenna argued in talks and books, as scientists today have gone into their study of matter and energy. These people—Taoist sages—meditated and felt time and determined it was describable not with ten or two hundred, or thirty or one hundred, but sixty-four parts, each with six subparts definable as yin or yang. With this knowledge, they created the *I Ching*, a 384-part system of time and accompanying text.

Three millennia later, at La Chorrera in 1971, when the mushroom was downloading a fractal model of time into McKenna's mind, McKenna asked why him. "You are the first person who has ever walked through this pasture who had these sixty-four hexagrams in your head," said the mushroom, a collagist. McKenna returned to the States and modeled the fractal wave in his Timewave theory on the oldest surviving yin-yang configuration—the King Wen sequence—for all 384 parts of the *I Ching*, whose structural correspondence with DNA he would call "staggering" in an interview in 1998, observing that all the processes in DNA, which expresses sixty-four codons, could be "easily modeled with the six line hexagrams."

While investigating the *I Ching*, which he called "the world's oldest book," McKenna also discovered it works—and was probably used in Neolithic China—as a lunar calendar. In *The Invisible Landscape*, he and his brother showed that an *I Ching* calendar, with thirteen lunations of 29.53 days totaling 383.89 days, resonated with sunspot cycles, zodiacal ages, and equinoctial precession and was more than twice as accurate as the solar, Gregorian calendar. In a lunar calendar, seasons slowly shift over years in a systematic sampling of possible variety. If winter began in December as a child, it would begin in August as a young adult; later in life, winter would again begin in December. Instead of stability and permanence, as with a solar calendar, the message of a moon-based calendar is gradual, constant, unceasing change.

18

On May 31, I emailed Kathleen Harrison—whose email address I'd gotten from her daughter, Klea, who I'd interviewed for Tao Of Terence—introducing myself and my book. "In the book's epilogue, I hope to write about you, Botanical Dimensions, the Ethnobotany Library which I'm eager to experience, and/or the drawing class I am excited to be taking from you and Paetra Tauchert on July 2," I said. I asked if we could talk for around an hour outside of the class. "If you'd rather not talk in this capacity, that is totally fine, and you don't need to provide a reason, I'll be able to write about the class and the library," I added.

19

In the fractal model of recovery that I began developing for personal use in 2013 and continue to ponder and use on myself, change becomes a kind of practice. A graph of fractal recovery from drugs and other problems is somewhat unpredictable in the short-term but stable and directional in the long-term. In fractal recovery, change happens to some degree in waves. Failure is expected and can be viewed partly as resonances of past failures, as unavoidable and useful and even enjoyable. Other strengths of the fractal model of behavior modification include that it has no rules so is optimized for creative involvement, that its main inspiration is nature (the longest surviving known system), and that it allows one to avoid ideology (rules coming from other humans) and so retain individuality even while making an earnest attempt at recovery. In my personalized model of fractal recovery, I've used these techniques:

- Note-taking. I've recorded, in notes.rtf, each time I've used a substance and the amount used. I've regularly studied my notes to learn and remind myself how much—and how—I've changed. By documenting life daily and scaling back to months and years to examine the past, I've generated momentum and confidence while increasing self-awareness and countering the distorting effects of memory.

- Busy isolation. Hiding in my room, I've refrained from entering situations that might cause anxiety, despair, and tedium that I'd want to ameliorate with the drugs I want to stop using. In my room, I've stayed productive and challenged by reading, writing, exercising, experimenting with psychedelics, and drawing extremely detailed mandalas.

- New worldview. I've immersed myself in a worldview almost the opposite of the bleak one I had before. I've done this by writing a column on McKenna—who I encountered in 2012 during the most problematic months of my "recovery"—and his ideas in 2014, and then in 2016 a book on my still-increasing interest in psychedelics and nature.

- New drugs. Instead of quitting all drugs—which still fascinated and excited me with their ability to selectively alter consciousness—I changed drugs. Encouraged by McKenna, who observed that drugs can be allies and that aboriginals have always used a variety of plant-based drugs, I shifted my drug interest from synthetic to natural, new to ancient.

20

Cannabis, the plant I've had the closest relationship with so far in my life, has been the main ally in my recovery. Early in our relationship, in August 2013, when I was in Australia for two book festivals, three weeks after throwing away my computer, I tweeted that I was seeking cannabis. A doctoral student named Oscar, who was studying if computers could write poetry, emailed me, met me in person, and gifted me cannabis that had been grown, he said, by the author of a book titled *Jesus Weed*. Oscar said cannabis made him both more judgmental and sensitive and I realized it did for me too.

I began smoking it daily the next month, in September, when my "recovery" ended. By then, I'd learned that my previous knowledge, absorbed from mainstream culture, on both drugs and psychedelics, had been wrong. And so instead of believing what seemingly everyone, even many who promoted it, said about cannabis—that it made one lazy, careless, paranoid, forgetful, and unproductive—I listened to Terence McKenna, Kathleen Harrison, and my own experiences and experiments with the plant and began to associate it with meticulousness, social interaction, physical activity, calmness, learning, empathy, wonder, creativity, and productivity.

In January 2014, I began to also eat cannabis, baked with coconut oil at 250 degrees in my oven for thirty minutes, once or twice a day. For months, then years, I occupied a new mental location where I accumulated feelings, ideas, habits, and memories. Stoned, I forgot what it felt like to be on Adderall or Xanax and so stopped being lured to them by my distorted memory of their effects. Instead of being only interminable, dreadful, and boring, my recovery, due largely to cannabis, which I looked forward to daily, was routinely exciting, educational, moving, and awe-instilling.

Stoned on ingested cannabis, I've felt back inside a dream I once had. Not like I was remembering it, but in it again, in its world, while also still in concrete reality, drawing a mandala. Stoned in bed, I've learned with amusement that an effect of a catalyzed imagination can be self-control; with my cannabinoided brain, automatically having more thoughts than normal, I once convinced myself to sleep by thinking of reasons why it was then the most desirable activity. I was surprised, as it happened, that it seemed to be working—I was pleasurably reasoning myself asleep.

21

On June 3, Kathleen responded she was "willing and interested to meet separately" from the class for a conversation. "I appreciate your tone, and I find the working title amusing," she said about my book, whose tone I'd called "positive and exploratory." After thinking it hundreds of times, I'd forgotten *Beyond Existentialism*, my book's then title, which twelve months later would become *Trip*, a suggestion by my publisher that attracted me for its dense minimalism, once seemed amusing to me too—in its "moving along now/then" indication of something being obviously past existentialism, which, in its assumption that the universe was indifferent and meaningless, seemed authoritatively like an end, not a phase. Kathleen mentioned I was probably referring by "beyond existentialism" to both the animist and the cosmic. In the animist worldview, every species was in conversation and humans were "just one of the beings," she'd said in her talk on cannabis. "We are a talking being," she'd observed with a smile. "And we really like to talk and we really like the illusion that we are the only ones talking."

22

On cannabis, alone in my room, thinking about family and friends and myself, remembering repressed and obscure and difficult and shameful moments, feeling compassion and self-pity and loneliness and joy and gratitude, I've sobbed and wept and profusely cried for, I estimate, ten to fifteen hours in 2013, 2014, and 2015. I've fallen down laughing for seemingly no reason, laughing uncontrollably on my hands and knees. I've often laughed for little, ridiculous, absurd, and unconscious reasons, reminding me I did this as a small child.

On cannabis I've spontaneously danced. I've intuited dance, something I normally never did or thought about, as a uniquely holistic activity, a behavior in which one tried, in a constantly evolving process, to relent to what each of the body's parts wanted—what amount and quality and configuration of contraction and relaxation, in what rhythm, at what speed, in which direction, would benefit it most and so feel most gratifying. I've felt dance as a behavior wanting to be done unconsciously. I've felt it as a yoga-like activity, dancing slowly while seated.

Cannabis has made exercise and stretching reliably engrossing, pleasurable, mentally stimulating, meditative, and a source of knowledge. Doing yoga on baked cannabis, I don't feel like I'm inside my body straining to push it into new positions, but, often, like I'm two large hands outside of myself, satisfyingly pulling my body into various shapes. Stretching stoned, I've realized that flexibility is like strength; in both, you increased the size of a muscle. In flexibility, a muscle became longer; in strength, thicker.

Cannabis transports me outside my sphere of worry—the dreary, unpleasant place where some to most of me normally exists and where, in my tetchiest moments, I feel unable to stop lingering on things I've already told myself to stop worrying about. Ingested carefully, before meaningful activities, cannabis can relocate all of me outside the sphere for more than three hours—often so far away I forget it exists. Smoked with strategic control of amount, timing, and purpose, cannabis transports me multiple times a day. Outside, I change my thoughts with surprising ease; instead of being distracted by my own worried face and recursive internal monologue, I see the world with unself-conscious, appreciative eyes.

23

On June 5, I responded that I was (referring to the animist and cosmic), that in my book I quoted McKenna on how nature wasn't mute but people deaf and that I planned to examine science fiction. I said I'd noticed that existentialism seemed to ignore "deep time"—that life had billions of years of history from which meaning and knowledge could be extracted, understood, and used. Something else I'd noticed about existentialism was that, for me, it had been partly a reaction to Christianity—the model of reality most people in Florida had used—which said to find meaning in the Bible. Existentialism, which said to make my own meaning, seemed more reasonable than Christianity. Similarly, the worldview McKenna had introduced to me (which sought meaning not from one book, oneself, or others but many books and people plus oneself, nature, and the unknown) seemed more reasonable—more curious and exploratory, including a larger context and so ignoring less information—than existentialism.

24

Cannabis has assuaged and underscored my degeneration. When moderately stoned, sometimes my teeth and gums ache in waves ranging from not unpleasant to mildly distracting and I can feel how my face is apparently always somewhat tensed and squished. When not stoned, parts of my face probably still feel vaguely numb, but over decades I've habituated, like others who've undergone years of torturous orthodontics to make their mouths presentable despite facial degeneration, to the sensation, absorbing it unknowingly into my personality and worldview.

By both soothing and sometimes gently alerting me to the existence of these and other pains, cannabis reminds me of a recommendation made by Arthur Schopenhauer in the nineteenth century, before degeneration worsened significantly in the twentieth and twenty-first centuries, that we greet one another not with "ma'am" or "sir" but, for accuracy and to remind us of "tolerance, patience, forbearance, and love of one's neighbor," "my fellow sufferer."

25

After two months in 1991 without cannabis, McKenna resumed smoking daily except while traveling and after his brain cancer diagnosis in May 1999. "At first I cut back on cannabis, because it seemed to trigger the seizures," he said in an interview in September 1999. "But then I easily got that corrected. Now I'm smoking as much dope as I ever did." In "Cannabis Trialogue," he wondered why he smoked so much. He answered because after writing for three hours and feeling depleted, he could smoke for "a second wind and a *third* wind to go forward with creative activity"; because it also revitalized him with physical work like stacking wood; because if he refrained, he worried about his "immediate short-term career goals," but if he smoked, he roved a world made of every book, person, and place he'd ever read, known, and been; and because if he refrained, his creativity was "a kind of brick-by-brick, linear extrapolation," but if he smoked, he could be surprised by "unexpected ideas."

26

On June 16, Kathleen responded to my June 5 email, offering dates for our conversation, including July 1, a Friday, and July 5, a Tuesday. I read her email at night in Bobst Library, then crossed the street into Washington Square Park, where, as I walked through, multiple people tried to sell me cannabis. Since arriving in New York in 2001, cannabis dealers in the park, concentrated usually in the northwest plaza, with more appearing at night, had unsuccessfully solicited my business probably more than two hundred times.

On June 18, walking to the library, I heard someone behind me on the sidewalk say, uncertainly, "No, I think whales know about humans." In the library, I thought about July 1 and July 5. I wasn't sure which to choose. I reread Kathleen's email and noticed she offered Friday first and that she'd mentioned a farmers market on Friday. I emailed her saying Friday would be good. She responded seventy-two minutes later, at 4:05 P.M., saying, "How about meeting me at the BD Library at 1pm," and that her son, Finn, who I'd also interviewed for Tao Of Terence, looked forward to meeting me.

The next day I noticed a ginkgo tree in Washington Square Park for the first time. My first time recognizing a ginkgo tree anywhere, by its unusual leaves, which I'd seen online, had been only two or three months earlier, by Gramercy Park; since then, I'd learned *Ginkgo biloba* was the only extant species in the Ginkgophyta division, which differentiated into class, order, and family Ginkgopsida, Ginkgoales, and Ginkgoaceae, and that the genus was at least two hundred million years old—around seven times older than cannabis and seventy times older than humans.

Now I was surprised to learn it lightly dominated the park—small ones like sleep-matted, jutting hair; large ones full and rising and Afro-like. Including one on the perimetering sidewalk, there were twenty ginkgo trees, concentrated in the southeast corner, across the street from Bobst Library, where I'd been 4,000 to 4,500 of the past 5,400 days. A tall, pagoda-shaped ginkgo shared the corner with the library and Goddard Hall, where I lived when I arrived in New York in fall 2001, when I took my first creative writing class and wrote poems about feeling sad, doomed, lonely, and meaningless.

27

I used to think there weren't that many species of life. There were the ones I saw on TV and in picture books—thousands, maybe. At some point I learned there were millions, which seemed like so many that hundreds or thousands going extinct seemed not disastrous. Now I felt there were barely any species, that each species was millions of years in a certain evolutionary direction, was like an explorer that had traveled through time in an unmapped direction and survived the dangerous journey to reach a place where it was alone and far away from everyone else, so that we had species like cannabis and salvia with their own unique compounds.

28

"We *are* a body of knowledge," said Kathleen in a talk given in 2010 in San Jose. "We are furthering it all the time through our brave and sometimes foolhardy investigations. And, so, what makes it research, then, is if we actually—individually—come out of each one of these investigations, these experiences, having learned something. Actually noting 'What did I learn?' and then doing your best to remember that—we know that that could be a challenge sometimes, but—adding that, then, to your body of knowledge. And part of the research, the value of it, then, is exchanging what you've learned with other people. So that's the 'telling the stories' part, you know. Telling the stories and the insights, 'cause the insights build on each other and they will continue to—they have over the years."

29

Kathleen's talks were created in front of their audiences, like in a meta, linguistic sport utilizing one's entire knowledge. This dynamic, practice-like method, which Terence also used but which otherwise seems somewhat rare, increased the complexity and relistenability of their talks while minimizing, for speaker and audience, redundancy and boredom. "I have not made a slideshow, I barely have any notes and I may not look at them, and I'm doing something that I seem to get more and more comfortable with as I age, which is I'm 'winging it,'" said Kathleen near the beginning of a talk on December 13, 2013, in San Francisco, eliciting laughter. "I . . . speak extemporaneously," she began a talk on a Sunday in summer 2015 in a sunny room at the University of Greenwich. "I gather my notes from my heart and my mind and the crowd and the event that I'm at. I challenge myself to do that."

30

In a profile of McKenna published in 1992 in *Esquire*, Mark
Jacobson wrote, "Immediately upon leaving Esalen, he drove like
a maniac to a gas station where he bought three Hershey bars
and a bag of Doritos." In the Q&A of "Plants, Consciousness, and
Transformation" (1995), McKenna said he'd been vegetarian "for
long periods" before. "Now I sort of follow the hippie philosophy that your body knows what it wants, even if it's a Snicker,"
he said, referring to Snickers bars, whose ingredients included
partially hydrogenated soybean oil, and laughed. On June 25,
1999, in a message to his mailing list nine months and nine days
before he died, McKenna discussed his cancer. He'd undergone
Gamma Knife surgery and was "having focused radiation treatments five days a week." He'd refused chemotherapy, which he
felt "may have to be tried if things get worse." He wrote:

> But my intuition is that the people who survive unusually
> long times are those who follow the surgery and radiation
> with extreme attention to cleaning up their diets and then
> supplement their diet very wisely. It is a wake up call to be
> very attentive to what goes into my body. You would think
> that an old psychonaut would have learned that long ago but
> what can I say? In other words attention to the details of food
> and nutrition will significantly prolong my life. How long?
> Who can say?

31

On the topic of worry, McKenna often referenced Wei Boyang, a second-century Taoist. When asked what he'd learned after a lifetime studying the *I Ching*, which viewed time as a finite number of irreducible elements like how the chemical elements composed matter, Boyang answered, "Worry is preposterous; we don't know enough to worry."

32

On June 20, in Bobst Library, I bought a round-trip ticket leaving for San Francisco on June 29, a Wednesday. I would arrive at night, travel to Occidental the next day, meet Kathleen on Friday, and be a student in her plant-drawing class on Saturday, I thought to myself. I would write about my experience. It would be the epilogue of my first nonfiction book.

33

In July, after returning from California and drafting the epilogue in first-person and changing it to third-person—to, among other reasons, explore what McKenna called "the main thing to understand," that we're "imprisoned in some kind of work of art"—I noticed someone in my peripheral vision moving toward me in small, robotic, slightly dance-like increments.

"Weed. Weed. Weed. Weed. Marijuana. Weed. Weed, weed, weed, weed," he said in a surprisingly loud, fast monotone, like a single-message Morse code. It was Sunday and I was walking through Washington Square Park, which was bustling—70 to 90 percent of seats occupied, people of all ages standing in sunlight—on my way to the library.

I briefly saw the man's hand, which displayed a plastic baggie of cannabis, underhand and proffering. This was the most conspicuously someone in the park had ever tried to sell me cannabis. But the offer didn't feel belligerent, being nonrhetorical and easily ignored, coming in a crowd in the form of a musical communication. I walked away smiling.

EPILOGUE

In Taoism, rest is a mere preparation for activity,
and death is but one stage in the transformation of Life.

—ELLEN MARIE CHEN

1. OCCIDENTAL

Twisting and pressing it with both hands in San Remo Hotel, Tao broke his computer's screen. He felt surprised and a little confused. It was June 29, 2016. He'd owned the computer since August 5, 2013, when he disposed of his previous one the morning after a solitary, post-midnight psilocybin trip. In the past year, he'd fixed its screen hundreds of times with his hands. Sometimes tens of slightly torqued squeezes, over minutes, were required to unfreeze the screen, yet he'd never felt at risk of breaking it, and now he'd cracked it on the second or third squeeze, easily and absently and distinctly as a knuckle. He suspected his unconscious—not unreasonably, he felt with interest and approval—for contributing to the "accident."

The broken screen looked like a painting of a segment of two-dimensional mountain, rising to the right at a 15-degree angle with 0- to 20-degree subangles, detailed with tiny trees and shrubs and grasses. A second slope, deliberate and lightly stylized as Chinese calligraphy, hovered above the left, lower side, so that the painting resembled a fractally embellished, runelike symbol of Kathleen Harrison's house, which also sloped acutely left, ended unexpectedly with two slopes, and was partially plant-covered.

Tao hadn't seen the house yet, so he didn't think of it as he posted a photo of the broken screen on Instagram. He'd handwrite this week, then, he thought—in the notebook he somewhat impulsively bought seven hours earlier by the Civic Center BART station, where many homeless people had milled. Tao had been in San Francisco in 2007, 2009, 2010, and 2013 to promote his poems, short stories, novella, and novels. Now he was there on his way to Occidental to meet Kathleen and be in her plant-drawing class, experiences he planned to model in his book's epilogue.

At 10:08 P.M., around fifteen minutes after cracking the screen, Tao emailed his mom from his iPhone asking about her mouth-doctor appointment, which he knew was the next day, because in May he'd noted it in notes.rtf—a file he'd typed 307,088 words in since October 28, 2013, when he created it to track his drug use, diet, sleep, exercise, and other behaviors against his mood. Sometimes he worried that his mom's jaw pain, which had begun in October 2015, might be advanced-stage cancer.

Sometimes he stopped himself from worrying, focusing instead on learning and on becoming a more encouraging and discerning and stable person—someone more able to help and console people, including himself, regardless of the situation. Tao didn't want to worry. He'd rather embody an always-evolving, performance-like behavior that was informed—not stifled or paralyzed—by his mental world.

But he'd already worried so much in his life. Worry comprised a major part of the finished object of himself—the five-or-more-dimensional object that, from somewhere outside time, was shareable and discussable and examinable as the text of a book was in time—and therefore he was susceptible, he felt, to worrying unconsciously. For the rest of his life, he could expect to sometimes become aware of himself worrying; these times, he would have the opportunity to stop.

In a FedEx Office the next morning, Tao printed a file of Kathleen-related information he'd collected, including excerpts of her talks, interviews, and essays. He rode BART to the airport. He lay supine on concrete in sunlight outside International Departures. He was there to ride the Airport Express bus to Santa Rosa. On his phone, he looked at photos from two months before he was born that had been recently posted online. "One of the few major psychedelics conferences during the dark age of the 'Just Say No' Reagan regime was the Psychedelics and Spirituality Conference (aka Psychedelic Conference II), held on the campus of UC–Santa Barbara on May 13–14, 1983," said text introducing the photos. Tao counted thirteen people in a photo in which Kathleen, seated in a chair, and Terence, below her on the floor, were looking at an old man who was bald. "We were the young ones in awe of the elders in 1983," said Kathleen's tweet linking the photos, taken when she was thirty-four and Terence was thirty-seven, via @BotanDim, whose profile said:

#Ethnobotany, plants, fungi, culture, food, native knowledge, healing, shamanism. Non-profit org, founded 1985 by Kathleen Harrison. Library, Classes & Festival

The traffic-prolonged three-hour bus ride to Santa Rosa passed quickly. In the front passenger-side seat, Tao enjoyed an aerial-seeming view of the road and bright scenery. He listened to a 1959 recording of Ann Schein playing a selection of Chopin études. He listened to a May 14, 2015, interview with Kathleen on a podcast called *Expanding Mind* in which she observed we all have indigenous ancestors, that for most of human history, immersed in nature, our worldview has been animist. "Basically right now I think we treat technology as the most animate engagement that we have with the world," she said. "If I may generalize about Western civilization," she added.

Passing Petaluma, Tao remembered his reading at a bookstore there in 2009, before his "recovery," "recovery"/recovery, recovery, and current mode, which was a kind of never-ending, practice-like recovery from most aspects of life as he'd experienced it so far—before all that. Two men had attended, one who resembled Salman Rushdie and didn't say anything, and a high school teacher interested in obscure punk/ska music. The latter, after the reading, drove Tao back to San Francisco, where they ate at a taco place. "We each have an observer," said Kathleen on *Expanding Mind*. "We can use that observer. We can engage that observer and carry her or him with each of us as we go." Near the end of the podcast, she said:

> *I* sometimes have to remind my*self*—I wobble in my balance, you know, with these elements—that there's a motivating spirit that's running through everything, and it takes many, many forms, endless forms and endless manifesta-

tions, whether it's life-forms or even idea-forms, thought-forms, and in some sense that's spirit. And it doesn't mean it's all good. That phrase, actually, sets me off. It's not "all good." Nothing is all good. But it's complex and beautiful and always changing, even with the suffering in it.

In Santa Rosa, Tao walked toward Whole Foods to eat and get a taxi to Occidental. He saw signs promoting Bernie Sanders for president. He imagined creating and carefully assimilating multiple "observers" into his unconscious, where they'd help him consider and maneuver his life. He thought about Santa Rosa's population of 174,170. Occidental's population, according to Wikipedia, was only 1,115 in 2010—around half to an eighth the number of Toba survivors, knew Tao, who in two weeks would read a book titled *Supervolcano* that argued the cataclysm trauma-tized the human species on a cellular level. On the bus his eyes had become watery from complex emotions five times. Now he felt focused and relaxed. Due to what he'd learned in the past two years about DNA and proteins and amino acids—information he'd eventually decide to include in his book as an appendix—he also felt enormous, bizarre, and that life pervaded the universe. It was late afternoon. Santa Rosa seemed quiet.

The idea to visit Kathleen first occurred to Tao sometime in fall 2014 when he wanted to convert his summer 2014 column, Tao Of Terence, into a small book by expanding it 20 to 30 per-cent and adding two chapters—"Life and Literature," on how life was like a higher-dimensional form of language-based art, and a chapter on Harrison, whom he'd regretted not devoting a post to in the column. He was glad that plan—which now seemed meager and strangely reluctant, as if he wanted to spend only a little more time, instead of the rest of his life, thinking about psychedelics and nature and the Mystery—hadn't happened.

Early in February 2016, after discussion with his editor, Tim, a McKenna fan since reading *Food of the Gods* as a teenager in the 1990s, Tao became excited about writing an all-new book, which would include only some of the column. He created an outline of the book that included an epilogue in which maybe he'd visit Kathleen in California. Tim approved of the outline and seemed especially interested in the epilogue, which Tao was further encouraged to actuate when he learned Kathleen was teaching a plant-drawing class on July 2, his birthday.

Days later, in mid-February, he began writing *Beyond Existentialism*, as his book was called then, based on a schedule that he and Tim both openly viewed as existing solely to help, not rush, him. In March, April, and May, he completed drafts of his book's introduction and first five chapters. He mostly successfully refrained from excessively worrying or fantasizing about the epilogue (how to collect material for it, what tone and form to use, if he should meet Kathleen or take the class but remain at a distance) and was able, he noticed with approval, to proceed with it gradually—buying the class ticket on April 22, emailing Kathleen on May 31, buying the plane ticket on June 20.

In June, while working on his book's cannabis chapter, Tao became a bit tired of Terence—in, he felt, an expected and healthy way, after four months immersed in his ideas. He'd had enough of Terence for now. He decided not to feature Terence's ideas in the chapter. As he experimented with structure, his notes on Kathleen's talk "Who Is Cannabis?" entered, roamed around, and eventually settled near the chapter's beginning. He welcomed Kathleen and her talk's subthemes—animism, cannabis as soothing ally, the histories of species, interspecies relationships—into the chapter, from where they would resonate, he knew, into the rest of the book, and on June 29, 2016, with around half his book written, he flew to San Francisco.

After checking into Occidental Hotel, Tao explored the small town, where his phone had no service, in late twilight. Occidental existed around a 0.6-mile stretch of a two-lane street called Bohemian Highway and had spacious sidewalks, a food store called Bohemian Market, a smaller food store, a restaurant called Hazel, an Italian restaurant called Negri's, Union Hotel, Sonoma Fine Wine, a café, a tavern, a bakery and juice bar, a volunteer fire department, a post office, a YMCA, and around ten other establishments. Houses were scattered throughout and on the overlooking, forested mountainsides.

Tao entered Harmony Village, which included apartments, a place for acupuncture and Chinese medicine, Occidental Center for the Arts, Botanical Dimensions's library, and an art gallery. Through a window briefly, Tao noticed more than ten, it seemed, elderly people drawing a naked woman. He slowly crossed the parking lot, toward houses with gardens, and incorrectly theorized Kathleen lived in one of them. The non-electronic, honkless, sirenless, vast-seeming peacefulness of his surroundings made him aware of himself, as a person, in the world.

His eyes suddenly teared up again, surprising him. He usually didn't cry this often. But his emotion was appropriate, he knew. He was doing something that, four years earlier, in 2012, he might've estimated a 1 to 3 percent chance of himself doing. Something rare was happening. He was here! The narrative of his life had led him to here—a place where he felt encouraged and surprised and moved by the story he was slowly experiencing. He walked a little more on Bohemian Highway to what seemed like the end of the town, then returned to the hotel on the other end, which was the south end.

In the hotel room, he emailed his friend Tracy saying he was meeting Kathleen the next day and felt "a little nervous." The email's subject was "Kathleen." He and Tracy had expressed admiration and interest in Kathleen and her work multiple times to each other. He emailed his mom, reread his Kathleen notes, and went outside to look at the stars, which he never saw in the city. He craned his head back and held it there in a strained motionlessness that was similar, he realized when it felt comically awkward, to how, since 2009 or 2010, he'd daily looked down to stare at phones. He couldn't specifically remember the last time he saw this many stars. The previous time, he'd also felt surprised, he vaguely recalled, by how small they made the universe seem. Now the stars also made the universe seem densely interconnected. Tao felt like he was looking at the stable, zone-like, pulsing insides of a thing.

In the past 10 percent or so of his life, he'd been contemplating and studying the possibility that the imagination, containing at least every imaginable universe, was infinitely larger than the universe, that dying released one into the imagination, and that the imagination was also where life itself, tunneling through matter on the surface of planets, was going—that a day, starting with morning and ending in dreams, was like a life, which was like life itself.

In the morning, Tao walked to a picnic bench and lay on it in warm sunlight. He felt sad and kind of doomed. Since February, he'd used 270 milligrams of caffeine within an hour, most days, of waking, and that day so far he'd used only around 20 milligrams, so his mood wasn't abnormal, but it felt abnormal and even troubling. He knew it was unreasonable and gullible to expect to always feel the same, but when he felt chemically depressed like this, the feeling sometimes too often tricked him into believing it was permanent. He remembered a recommendation by Kathleen on *Expanding Mind*, to "spend two minutes looking at a single leaf" when one felt "self-obsession of some sort." He lifted his body, removed a leaf from a tree, and returned to a supine position. The fractal leaf, backlit by sunlight, reminded him of the fractal nature of recovery—that he'd feel better in the long-term but not always in the short-term.

Back in the hotel room, Tao read an email from his mom, who'd gone to the mouth doctor that morning. The doctor had prescribed a "mouth guard" after diagnosing her with protruding bones on both sides of her mouth. "So nothing serious, don't worry," said Tao's mom in summary and conclusion. Historically above-average worriers, Tao and his mom often told and reminded—and sometimes requested and, saying "please," even pleaded with and beseeched—each other and themselves not to worry. Tao didn't dwell on his gladness that it wasn't cancer; he'd automatically feel the effect of the news, he knew, over hours and days and weeks, like a complex time-release pill. He was glad the doctor hadn't tried to prescribe a drug.

2. KATHLEEN HARRISON

Tao photographed the note, dated 12:54 P.M., on the library door from Kathleen saying she'd be back in ten minutes, then walked around talking to himself—a complex, multipurpose tool he'd avoided at times in the past in part, he suspected, due to society's dim view of it, associating it with complete insanity or a kind of neurotic mindlessness. The behavior seemed especially stimulating and valuable and sanity-helping for Tao, who often spent his time in mute aloneness. He wondered aloud what to do about recording. He'd recently become conflicted about whether to record part, all, or none of his formal and/or informal interactions with Kathleen. As he talked to himself, Tao realized with some surprise—which made him aware part of him had been pessimistically anticipating he'd realize nothing useful—what he'd say.

He practiced saying it and it made sense and he felt capable. Sometimes his intuitions while stoned seemed powerful and lucid at first but upon examination became dull and strangely vague, but not, it seemed, this time; as he became more familiar with this state of consciousness, his discernment within it increased. He was caffeinated and cannabinoided to feel at his most social and curious and lively and charming, his least troubling and joyless. In the past, this required not-small amounts of benzodiazepine, amphetamine, and caffeine; afterward, he'd feel terrible, suicidal. Now it could be achieved on low to moderate amounts of caffeine, smoked cannabis, and ingested cannabis; afterward, he often felt pleasantly tired and existentially reinvigorated.

Kathleen had parked in the distance and, obscured by cars, was approaching. Tao began recording a Voice Memo, which he'd stop and delete if they, in a few minutes, decided against recording, as per his just-conceived plan. He thanked Kathleen for meeting him and for her note and its specificity. He said his mom was also specific to the minute in handwritten notes.

They entered the library, a rectangular room around the size of Tao's apartment, and discussed Huichol art on a wall. The peyote-using Huichols had lived in the mountains of central Mexico for at least 15,000 years, according to carbon dating of ashes in their fireplaces, and now lived in western Mexico. Kathleen offered Tao a pair of plant parts to smell. His hands trembled like faceless animals as he held the plants, which smelled like sage. He said his parents' toy poodle enjoyed rolling around in sage, meaning, though, he'd realize months later, rosemary.

Kathleen asked where they lived.

Tao said Taipei. He said since they were going to move around—and not just sit, like he imagined Kathleen might've imagined when he asked, in his May 31 email, if they could talk for an hour—he wanted to ask again how she felt about being recorded. Kathleen said she felt fine.

Tao said he'd rather not record if it would make anyone self-conscious.

Kathleen asked if it would make Tao self-conscious.

"No," said Tao, feeling a little self-conscious.

Kathleen said it wouldn't make her self-conscious, either.

Tao said good and disengaged the "try to remember" and note-taking parts of himself. He chose a yerba maté from the library's large selection of teas—gifts from "tea people"—and said he didn't talk much and encouraged Kathleen to talk about anything for as long as she wanted.

Kathleen said two conferences had invited her to give talks on, specifically, tobacco. Tao said he'd noticed and liked Kathleen's fondness for tobacco. She asked why. Thinking of how most people associated tobacco with corporations, lies, cigarettes, and cancer instead of the genus of plant, which aboriginals had chewed, smoked, insufflated, used as an ingredient in ayahuasca, and drunk as a cold-water infusion for millennia in its naturally pesticide-and-additive-free form, Tao said because it was different and unexpected. He said he was currently writing his book's chapter on cannabis and that it included notes on Kathleen's talk "Who Is Cannabis?," which he'd listened to around five times. Kathleen asked if Tao was a "cannabis person" and realized she already knew he was, from Twitter. Tao praised Kathleen's writing, citing her precise, concise prose and interestingly varied sentence structures. She thanked him for the feedback and said the latter wasn't conscious. He learned she'd published an essay on "tripping in nature" in a Multidisciplinary Association for Psychedelic Studies newsletter.

Kathleen brought the teas to the table, which was between tall bookshelves. Tao momentarily believed the notepad and pen on the table were for him, then admired Kathleen's preparedness, then identified a framed piece on a wall as by Klea McKenna. It was from *Rainstorms & Rain Studies, 2013–2016*, her "ongoing series of unique gelatin silver photograms of rain made outdoors at night," according to her website, which showed twenty-three from the series. In the first, rain droplets containing their own shadows resembled elongated, blurrily falling birdcages. The fourth seemed to Tao like an aerial, computer-enhanced view of the different-size forms of life in a randomly selected rectangle of nature; it was all dots, from tiny and blobby to even tinier and pixel-like; as little as the blobs were, the pixels seemed hundreds to thousands of times littler.

They sat facing each other. Tao had at other times considered that maybe the questions he'd prepared would be background information—that, finally, he wouldn't use them—and now he felt sure of this. He wouldn't try to ask his questions. He would try to inconspicuously and somewhat slyly encourage Kathleen to talk about whatever she wanted to talk about that day.

———

Kathleen Harrison was born on August 12, 1948, on Catalina Island, around twenty-two miles off the coast of Los Angeles. She was the eldest of three siblings, with two younger brothers. Her parents divorced when she was fifteen. When she was sixteen, her dad said, "I think you might be a 'bohemian.' Do you know what a bohemian is?" She said she did. She said she too thought she might be one.

She learned of psychedelics from her mom, who took LSD with a Maori woman who lived with their family when Kathleen was a teenager. Her mom didn't tell her about LSD. Rather, one day Kathleen found a piece of paper with handwriting by her mom that began legibly and ended in scribbles.

At the University of California, Santa Cruz, she studied art and phenomenology. She was open to trying almost anything. She called herself an "experience junkie."

In Jerusalem in 1967, her best friend, Nina, introduced her to Terence. Kathleen recognized him from a dream the previous night. She'd been walking along a cliffside. Terence had approached and they'd passed each other, edging by, and then Kathleen saw an island in the distance and wondered why it was in silhouette. Terence, in concrete reality, said he was on his way to the Seychelles to live on Silhouette Island. "You're a good dreamer," he told Kathleen. They met again one spring eight years later, moved to Hawaii that fall, and married the following fall.

Kathleen said Terence wanted marriage but she didn't, and Tao asked why. "I think he thought," said Kathleen, then explained that maybe Terence—who otherwise avoided many modern institutions, for example not keeping his money in banks—had thought marriage would tame him, keep him focused. Kathleen said she felt marriage could actually do the opposite. She said maybe Terence wanted to exhibit some normality to his family. She added with a smile that she enjoyed "a good ironic reversal."

They moved to Freestone—a town by and even smaller than Occidental—where they knew no other people. They created a mail-order company called Lux Natura in 1977 to sell *Psilocybe cubensis* spore prints. Finn was born in 1978, Klea in 1980, both at home. Kathleen's "experience junkie" lifestyle ended; she focused on nursing her children for six years, during which she refrained from tripping—imperfectly, she qualified with a smile, which Tao reciprocated widely. Every day, Terence woke at 6:00 A.M., swept the floor, made a pot of coffee, began smoking hash—the same every day.

Tao asked if Kathleen was like that.

"Me?" she said. "No. I like variety."

She called Terence a narcissist, then a few sentences later connected him with a history of "brilliant narcissists." She observed this didn't make him a good husband or father. She said he used to smoke cannabis heavily—when it was illegal even medically—in the house's central location, where their children sometimes played with friends. This stopped when they built a loft for smoking in at the top of the house. Every night, Kathleen and Terence met there and talked.

After it became illegal to sell *Psilocybe cubensis* spore prints, Lux Natura began selling psychedelics-related art and essays and also audiotapes and transcripts of Terence's talks, which for years he'd practiced exclusively on Kathleen, who helped him develop and hone the style of lecturing he later used for almost two decades to share ideas with people. The "someone" referenced by Terence in his 1993 *tripzine* interview who persuaded him to speak publicly about psychedelics was Kathleen.

Discussing Terence's work, Kathleen said *The Invisible Landscape* was unreadable. She reiterated the book was unreadable and Tao grinned and the grin became a large smile. She said there was a time when Terence said things like "If people can't understand what I'm saying, they don't deserve to know my ideas" and that she'd convinced him otherwise. Which led to *True Hallucinations*, which had originally been titled *Down to Earth*. Kathleen had suggested *True Hallucinations*. Tao said he much preferred *True Hallucinations* because *Down to Earth* reminded him of the idiomatic expression meaning practical, ordinary, and wholesome.

He asked Kathleen about her writing. What did people want to read by her? She said people had expressed interest in reading her account of her and Terence's 1976 trip to the Amazon. Tao asked how she felt about "Among *Ayahuasqueros*," Terence's account. Kathleen said she'd been Terence's editor through the 1980s, and the essay, first published in 1989 in the anthology *Gateway to Inner Space*, "got through": she'd approved of it, but that, still, it was only his side of the story.

She said people had also wanted to read her account of an episode at the end of *True Hallucinations* in which, on psilocybin in Hawaii with Terence, she encountered a vehicle with entities in it that began to beam her up—UFO-style—but weren't successful. Tao said he vaguely remembered that scene. Kathleen said she hadn't read any of Terence's books since their breakup twenty-five years earlier. She shared her account of the trip, which she'd written in a journal; she'd felt like the entities wanted her because she'd learned something she wasn't supposed to know.

As Kathleen discussed UFOs, explaining they were viewed differently in the 1970s and 1980s than now, there was a cough that seemed twenty to thirty feet away. Kathleen said it was an accountant on the other side of the wall and wondered if he could hear her and Tao talking about UFOs and LSD. She warned Tao there was also a dog, which might bark, and later it did—once, at a moderate volume, like in a roll call of attendance.

Tao learned Kathleen smoked cannabis around four nights a week and that, in addition to her cannabis-inspired journal, which filled twenty notebooks and was handwritten at night, she kept a journal on her computer that was typed in daytime on coffee. Tao said he'd heard Terence, in a trialogue on cannabis, say that when he abstained from cannabis for two months, he read more and his dream-life became more interesting but he was otherwise unaffected. Kathleen said he'd been miserable and overbearing, with seemingly no sense of humor, those months—a nightmare to be around, for her and their children—and Tao smiled, amused.

At one point, Kathleen said she'd always just gotten by, financially, and Tao remembered his own career—$500 to $1,500 advances on his first six books, working in a restaurant, selling shoplifted batteries on eBay. He mentioned *Nutrition and Physical Degeneration* at one point, and Kathleen wrote the title on her notepad. He asked if her children had braces. She said no but maybe should have—Finn had a crooked bite. Tao expressed his opinion that it was good they hadn't. He mentioned his tongue being too big for his mouth, his eight pulled teeth.

Two other dialogues occurred while in the library. Klea called and talked to her mom for a few minutes, then Finn texted and Kathleen said he was at the house and would like to meet Tao. As a joke, Tao said he thought Kathleen was going to say that Finn had texted to say he was coming now to bring Tao some cannabis.

Kathleen said that could be arranged. Tao thanked her and then talked about something else. Seated in the quiet room, he felt maybe both a little overcaffeinated and a little overcannabinoided. Sometimes, during their conversation, he'd partially to fully lost track of what was being discussed, but this seemed okay since his phone was recording.

Kathleen was surprised it was already 3:00 P.M. She'd said she was free until 4:00 P.M., Tao knew, and they hadn't walked and talked yet. She'd said, in an email, that she "loved walking-talking in nature." They decided to visit her garden, which surrounded her house.

After they stood, Tao said he did better when not sitting and staring at the other person, then realized he'd said something probably better suited—more comprehensible and relevant—for his internal monologue. Photographing a bookshelf, he unwittingly stopped the Voice Memo. He photographed more bookshelves, thinking he'd read the titles from the photos later.

Kathleen's car's dashboard, lightly strewn with dried plant matter, reminded Tao of his low table where he'd been working significantly more with plants in the past half year—maintaining two or more syncopated fermentations, routinely buying new plant parts from the farmers market in Union Square to taste, eat, smoke, smell, burn, chew, dry, photograph, collect, and draw. Kathleen parked in her driveway by peach trees. She opened the passenger door, which didn't open from inside, then rapidly felt around fifteen peaches until finding one suitably ripe for Tao, who idly felt four or five that all seemed similarly ripe. One thing he'd forgotten to praise about Kathleen's writing was the range and amount and density of information, emotion, and life it conveyed. Her essay in *Sisters of the Extreme* began with this seven-sentence paragraph:

I had grown the plant—*Salvia divinorum*—for twenty years, and I knew the scant botanical and anthropological literature on this rare, sacred plant, but I'd never successfully had a visionary experience from ingesting the leaves. Once I'd tried putting thirty leaves in a blender with water and drinking the green slurry, but other than a headache and distinct empathy with a trapped butterfly, not much had happened. In the summer of 1995 I was ready for another in my series of solo ethnobotanical fieldwork adventures, and so I headed off for a month in the mountains of northern Oaxaca, Mexico. My son and daughter were staying with family, and I had work to do: not only investigating the folk uses and beliefs regarding healing plants, but also a health challenge of my own. For a couple of years following the dissolution of my marriage and the sad, slow death of my father, my heart had not been beating regularly. I'd always had a heart murmur and the strain of recurrent anemia, but this was more disturbing, grabbing my breath away. After one episode with a doctor, I decided I wanted to ask a Mazatec healer to do a ceremony for me with the Leaves of the Shepherdess.

Peach in hand, walking downslope on her driveway, Tao asked Kathleen what the doctor in her essay had told her. To take medication that would be for the rest of her life, she answered.

Tao said he'd been trying to keep his parents away from non-holistic doctors—a group that had historically prescribed them symptom-treating, cause-ignoring, destructive drugs—and teach them to focus on diet, which doctors learned little about in school. According to a paper published in the *American Journal of Clinical Nutrition* in 2006, medical school students in the United States in 2004 received, on average, only 23.9 hours of nutrition instruction—which the paper called "inadequate," Tao knew. Kathleen added "exercise" and Tao said "diet and exercise," agreeing. He'd forgotten exercise. Doctors did encourage exercise.

"Wow," said Tao when he saw Kathleen's house, a wooden triangle surrounded by a diverse variety of plants, including tall trees.

They entered Kathleen's somewhat L-shaped garden, toward an end with a cottage. Tao said he was seeing plants he hadn't seen before and Kathleen encouraged him to take photos, film movies. She gave him a tour of the narrow cottage, where Klea and her husband and their daughter were staying currently. Tao said it was a little bigger than his room in New York. He exited the cottage, saw Finn, and said, "I'm Tao."

On the phone with Klea in the library, Kathleen had pronounced his name Dao; now in the garden he explained to her and Finn that he pronounced it Tao and that in Florida, where he grew up, most people, unfamiliar with the philosophy, had called him Tay-O; some had called him Towel.

In Mandarin, each syllable could be said in four tones, each with at least one symbol and meaning—妈 (mā), 麻 (má), 马 (mǎ), and 骂 (mà) meant "mom," "numb" or "cannabis," "horse," and "scold," for example. Tao's name, 韬/Tāo, was unrelated to the Tao or Dao, 道/Dào, of Taoism. Despite asking his mom every few years, Tao had never been able to confidently remember what his name meant. It had something to do with hiding and jade, about hiding then appearing and succeeding, or something.

There'd been a time when, for reasons he'd forgotten, Tao believed his name did refer to Taoism. During that time, for months or years, he'd avoided Taoism despite feeling attracted to its ideas because he didn't want to be interested in something that was his name, which he didn't choose. He was glad his name meant something else—"Your Tao (韬) is usually in a phrase called 韬光养晦 (hiding and cultivating the jade like shining good in order to shine someday)," said his mom in one email as her entire explanation. That his name didn't refer to Taoism increased Tao's interest in Taoism. "While the Greeks worshipped strength and beauty of form, Taoism considers the grotesque and deformed and weak somehow to belong more to the process of change, thus they are closer to the Mother," wrote Ellen Marie Chen in a 1974 essay that began with an observation Tao hadn't heard before: "One important aspect of thought in the *Tao Te Ching*, the significance of which has so far been neglected, is its emphasis on the feminine."

Tao had learned of Chen from Merlin Stone, whom he'd encountered through the Goddess religion, which he'd learned about from Riane Eisler, whom he'd heard of from Terence McKenna, who'd also introduced him to Kathleen Harrison.

Kathleen showed Tao a plant whose leaves had looked completely insect-eaten from a distance. The plant wasn't goldenseal but contained the 43-atom compound berberine like goldenseal.

Finn introduced two Panamanian tobacco plants. Tao touched a large, soft, lime-green trichomed leaf. He held another leaf to it and they cohered as if tinily Velcroed. "I've never seen cannabis," he said as a partial non sequitur.

Kathleen said it was tobacco they were gathered around.

Tao said he had not seen cannabis or tobacco in person.

Kathleen said Finn was a bit obsessed with gardening and Finn said it wasn't a bad thing to be obsessed with and Tao thought of a character in a novel he'd read in April who'd collected "petascale volumes" of pornography. In his research, Tao had sometimes encountered the question of how Amazonian aboriginals found two plants out of tens of thousands to combine to achieve orally active DMT. People seemed somewhat baffled by this, but Tao felt it made sense. How, after all, had Japanese players of Super Mario Bros. learned to access 256 secret levels

by removing the cartridge without turning off the system, insert-
ing the unrelated game Tennis, playing it a little, and reinserting
Mario? By being obsessed, curious, and exploratory. Living outside history for at least 265,000 years, aboriginals had been more
interested and involved in plants, Tao estimated, than twentieth-
century people in Nintendo.

Kathleen indicated an area where Finn used to play as a child.

Tao misidentified red chard as beet, then identified lacinato
kale—in the distance, dark green. Kathleen referenced its blue-
ness, which Tao then noticed. He looked at a sloped, pathless
area dominated by feverfew, a knee-high, white-flowered plant
that grew throughout the garden in a pleasingly random-seeming
manner. He photographed and touched cannabis, which seemed
a more conspicuous green than the other plants, almost neon.

The fractal garden and triangle house thrived, Tao felt, on the
craggy, almost mountainously sloped, modest-to-small property. Due to the many curvy paths Kathleen had allowed to
naturally develop, the garden seemed large and immersive and
explorable—a place with many of its own special places. Tao consciously, subconsciously, and unconsciously imagined the garden in the form, among others, of a text-based computer game,
a 16-bit role-playing game, a nonlinearly fragmentary essay, and
a nonfiction book. He began talking, at some point, about turmeric. He said he'd recently—six months earlier—learned he
had ankylosing spondylitis, an autoimmune disease causing
inflammatory pain in his hips and back that turmeric relieved.

Kathleen asked how much turmeric he ate.

Tao didn't know what to say.

Kathleen said she was curious because she also ate turmeric.

Sensing, somewhat uncertainly, that she was talking about

turmeric in its powdered form, Tao felt self-conscious. He didn't want to seem "more hard-core," some part of him thought, than Kathleen by revealing how much whole, raw, powdered, boiled, and fermented turmeric he ate; he also didn't want to, because it seemed ridiculous to lie about this. Vaguely, without eye contact, he said something like "I just eat a piece sometimes" and felt rude and closed off. He looked away and felt disappointed in himself and confused—he wouldn't formulate a theory on why he'd suddenly lied until examining this situation later in prose—but then recovered almost instantly from the convoluted faux pas that now seemed okay and at least partially amusing. He reminded himself he lived in relative hermitude and that his brain and mind were broken in thousands to millions of ways, that his temporary malfunction wasn't unexpected. It was expected and so could be meta-experienced and, in various ways, enjoyed.

Tao said turmeric, which contained anti-inflammatory curcuminoids, had helped him a lot. He felt less pain and suppler since he began eating it daily in January. For the first 95 percent of his life, chronically inflamed and swollen, he'd never been able, for example, to crack his knuckles—it had seemed strangely impossible. He'd felt confused by his peers who casually and seemingly enjoyably—were they just stronger and/or braver and/or more pain-tolerant?—squeezed their fingers to produce unexpectedly loud, satisfying-sounding noises. Now he cracked his knuckles and other joints often, with physical and intellectual pleasure, as a technique to further differentiate his body and to test what its thousands of parts felt like—and could do—at different times on different days on different drugs and foods. Pushing, pulling, arranging, and stretching it into positions new to him but not his species, Tao regularly heard and felt his body emit pleasing and informative sounds.

Kathleen used the word "hospitality," which made Tao antici-
pate beverages or snacks, then asked if he'd like some cannabis.

Facing the garden and the grapevine-covered back of the house,
they sat by a shed and smoked cannabis—except Kathleen, who
refrained. Tao looked at tens of species—in pots on the railing
and hanging from the ceiling—on a second-floor covered bal-
cony. Finn offered him a hash-and-tobacco joint. After smoking
one hit, Tao felt very different. It seemed the opposite of bleak to
him that people had the opportunity in life to significantly modulate their cannabinoid systems for the first time—and that one
could refrain for hours, days, or years and do it again, the effect
recharged by time. He looked at tiny green grapes. He looked
at Oriental poppy pods resembling intricate models of massive,
fantastical structures. Like feverfew, various species of poppy
grew throughout the garden. They'd stood at some point—and
Kathleen had gone inside—and now they sat again on the edge
of the garden.

Tao expressed interest in living in the cottage on the other
side of the garden. Finn smiled and seemed to like this idea. He
said if Tao wanted a place to "hermit out," there would be good.
In the past few months, Tao had sometimes considered just moving to Occidental—"just" because he knew he wanted to move
to California but wasn't sure where exactly—but the possibility
of living in Kathleen's garden hadn't occurred to him. Finn said
he'd tell his mom he approved of Tao potentially renting the cottage when/if it became available.

After Kathleen returned with cups of mildly sweet, effer-
vescent drinks, Tao told her and Finn about his book. The first
chapter was on encountering Terence in 2012, the second was a

biography of Terence, the third was on Tao's drug history, fourth on psilocybin, fifth on DMT, sixth on cannabis (which would later become eighth), seventh on salvia, and eighth on why psychedelics were illegal. Tao described three more chapters—which he would write in the next six months to complete a first draft of the book and then, after receiving Tim's purifying edits, absorb into the second and third drafts as fragments, sentences, and passages—and said the book's epilogue would be about meeting Kathleen, and Finn, and the drawing class the next day.

Finn, smiling in a way that calmed and pleased Tao, said he looked forward to reading the book. He said he was amused their "little plant-drawing class" might be "a snippet" in a book that would be read by intellectuals and literary people in New York— "the literati." Tao was amused and stimulated by Finn's amusement. He wasn't sure what Finn's conception of that group of people was, but he guessed something like severely disconnected from nature, atheist, cynical, pessimistic, and depressed. Without thinking of anyone, Tao said he wanted to convert "those people," his readers, worldview-wise, with his book. Then he said he was just living his life, taking a plant-drawing class, that actually the book was secondary.

Kathleen asked how he became interested in writing.

Tao talked about shyness.

Kathleen asked his age.

Tao said thirty-two, and then they discussed Botanical Dimensions, which had been created when Tao was one or two. Kathleen asked if Tao knew BD's origin story. Tao said he'd heard it in one of her talks but would like to hear it again; compared to her prose, which seemed chiseled and somewhat geometric, Kathleen's spoken language, in her talks, was curving and jutting and gently flailing and organistic and unpredictable, often producing unusual, unlikely-to-be-written sentences. Tao had heard the story in the Q&A of her December 13, 2013, talk, in which she shared how, one night long ago, seated in a circle during an ayahuasca ceremony with "a couple of beloved troopers," she'd gotten up, gone outside, sat, and looked at the stars.

> And I saw this human heart—not a classic heart but a human heart—way, way, way out there in space, with ribbons blowing in the breeze off of it, and I was just like, "Really, the human heart way out in space; now that is really interesting." So I was at a moment in my life where, because my kids were just old enough that I thought now I could just really seize what my work is in the world—and I haven't said it yet, but that's always been much of my question: "What is my work? What is my work for the next stretch of the path? I don't need to know the whole picture all the way for the rest of my life. I'd just like to see to the place that the path turns again, please." And, so, I asked that question and the answer was, from ayahuasca and the spirit, I felt: "Put the plants front and center." And I had just seen this huge human heart and I was, you know, on ayahuasca, and I was struck by the power and the beauty of that for a moment, and then I said: "You're a plant; of course you're going to tell me to put the plants front and center! I have two small children. I have to put *them* front and center." And it was like, "Well, okay, behind the children—no more negotiating."

Botanical Dimensions was founded in 1985. Kathleen and Terence bought land in Hawaii and Terence raised money through his name and people all over the world mailed them plants and not all survived but some did and these were planted in the Ethnobotanical Forest-Garden, BD's eight-acre botanical repository. Kathleen had planted twigs that were now big trees.

She said that when Terence left BD, after their divorce in 1992, he "basically took 'the talking part' with him" and that she kind of regretted spending so much time helping him with his talks instead of working on her own projects, which included teaching since 1991, almost-annual fieldwork with the Mazatec since 1994, writing a collection of essays since 2007, the Amazonian Digital Herbarium Project since 2010, BD's internet presence since 2013, and now BD-sponsored classes, workshops, and events—including the first Ethnobotany Festival & Symposium in eleven weeks—and the new library, which opened on November 14, 2015.

Tao said but now it was bringing people like him to her.

Kathleen smiled and said people had so far been willing to come to Occidental for classes and events. Tao said she deserved it after all her work. He asked what had been in the room before the Ethnobotany Library. Kathleen said the room had been too big for anyone to want to rent and now half was the library, containing her and donated books, and half was the accountant and his dog. "This is how it should be," she said about her garden having many species together.

"This is how I would want my garden to be if I had one," said or thought Tao, becoming increasingly stoned. He remembered a moment in Kathleen's writing, which he began praising again. He'd felt surprised and moved by Kathleen's description of metaphysical transportation, finding herself "in another realm, astonished" while chewing salvia leaves. Tao said he'd only smoked salvia as dried leaves with extract added.

Kathleen said if he moved to California he could try the fresh leaves. Tao thanked her and said he'd like that. She reconfirmed with Finn to supply him with cannabis for later. Tao said he'd brought some dry cannabis and also capsules of baked cannabis. Kathleen said she'd made olive oil tinctures in the past for travel, then went in her house. She had first smoked DMT in pure form, Tao knew, in 1975—an experience she described in 2010 as filled with "more information in a shorter time that was retrievable than I have ever experienced before or since."

Tao told Finn that, in New York, he hung out with a person only once a week, or less, and Finn said something like "I prefer to live in the woods myself." Tao said this was the only time he'd left New York to do something that wasn't a book tour or parent visit or family vacation, but something he'd conceived and planned himself. He said he usually stayed home. He'd imagined Kathleen and/or Finn imagining him writing one of those nonfiction books in which the author visits someone new in every chapter, asking them questions they've already answered in their work. Tao tried to abstain from those questions because they usually led, for him at least, to redundant answers that were less clear and accurate than he'd already meticulously expressed in context in print; it felt a little petulant to ask people to repeat themselves in different words just for his book.

For his book, Tao was only visiting Kathleen. His book would trend toward the feminine, he'd begun to think. In conveying evolution over years of a life, it would itself evolve a little, from yang to yin, dead to alive, Terence to Kathleen.

Tao and Finn discussed the plant-drawing class, which Finn was attending as a student. Tao had posted two pieces of Finn's art with his interview with Finn for Tao Of Terence and both had shown teeth. They'd also included a face with a smaller face on its forehead, a cartoon figure half the size of the face, two two-headed entities (one with a nongeometric body sprouting geometric mazes), and an area of straight-angled lines morphing dimensionally into beings of various ontological status. Finn explained that his visual art wasn't plant-focused, but that the next day's class still interested him, though his art wasn't averse, either, to plants.

"You're not changing your direction," said Tao in summary.

Finn laughed in a way that made Tao want to make him laugh more.

"I'm not changing my direction," he confirmed.

Kathleen came outside, ready to drive to the library.

Walking to her car, they discussed a benefit event thirteen days earlier—for Botanical Dimensions and the Green Earth Foundation—featuring Kathleen and Ralph Metzner in "a conversation between two old friends." In an email the day after the event, Kathleen had mentioned it'd gone "very well," though Metzner had been "rather ponderous in mood and content." Finn said Metzner had railed against the idea of the double-blind study, then said something that Tao uncertainly interpreted as meaning Metzner had bristled in some way when Kathleen, during the conversation, spoke of myths as metaphors. Ahead of Tao and Finn, Kathleen said, "I think I said science was a metaphor," which Tao quickly emailed himself to contemplate later; his phone had no internet connection in the garden but the email would go through later, he knew.

By then, he'd stopped recording audio. While talking to Finn around an hour earlier, he'd noticed his phone had stopped recording—around when, he calculated, he and Kathleen left the library. He'd been excited to be recording their informal interactions (in the car, on the driveway, in the cottage and garden) but apparently he hadn't been, he realized with disappointment, then started a second Voice Memo, then minutes later noticed he'd, again, unintentionally stopped recording—by photographing, he finally realized. He then recorded a third, brief Voice Memo—to sample Finn's peculiar, difficult-to-remember language—after which, around a half hour earlier, he committed to stop recording for the day.

Opening her car door, Kathleen said Metzner might've been suffering that night from age-related pain, which made him depressed. She said she could relate.

"I can relate to that also," said Tao over the car. "I feel depression . . . often."

"You and I have felt physical pain," said Kathleen in the car, looking at Tao in the passenger seat. She said it could be hard. Combined, Finn, who was in the back seat, and Tao were seventy years old, two years more than Kathleen.

Looking ahead through the windshield, Tao said that, after suspecting for around a decade that his hip-and-back pain was due to a macrophysical problem, like a herniated disc or pectus excavatum—a degenerative deformity he had that affected ten to eighty in one thousand people, making their chests sunken in front—he'd learned in January that it was probably mostly microphysical, involving compounds and microorganisms. Now that he knew, he could help himself with diet. Kathleen asked how. Giving the simplest formulation, Tao said by avoiding starches. "By eating more like our aboriginal ancestors," he later realized he could've said.

During the drive to Harmony Village, where Kathleen would meet Paetra to prepare for the following day's class and Finn and Tao would walk to the farmers market, Tao asked Kathleen how the Mazatec found *Salvia divinorum* and she said she didn't know that story. The Mazatec always told her, even when she asked more than once, that they'd known whichever plant forever—even coffee, which they began growing around 1850, and tobacco, which was introduced to them one to five thousand years ago.

Outside the library, Tao met Paetra, who had a calmly alert demeanor that encouraged him to skip small talk. "I heard you've never taught before," he said, feeling encouraging and interested, then realized he'd exceeded something maybe, then realized it was okay when Paetra said, in amicably gameful response, "I heard you're thinking of moving to Northern California."

Tao was peripherally aware of the route's idiosyncratic form—the result, he imagined, of thousands of cross-town walks—as he and Finn walked to the farmers market. His caffeine (iced coffee before and yerba maté in the library) and nicotine (from Finn's joint) had worn off. The cannabis capsule he swallowed two hours before meeting Kathleen had worn off. But the hash and cannabis he smoked in the garden were still helping him and so he felt in a good mood, laughing and speaking often.

But then at some point he began to suspect his laughter might be disconcerting, inappropriate, offensive, or disturbing. He realized he'd laughed—maybe loudly, as if at an unexpectedly funny joke—after Finn said his "thirty-five-year-old friend" who'd recently undergone hip surgery would be in the class the next day. But it hadn't been a joke. Finn had been directly answering a question about who else would be in the following day's class. Tao wasn't sure—and, in the confusion, didn't ask—why Finn, who seemed to ignore his laughter, had focused specifically on his friend's age, saying "thirty-five-year-old" before anything else. Finn was thirty-eight. How was thirty-five significant? Had he misheard something?

After that, Tao became quiet and humorless, losing his sense of tone and long-term purpose. His voice now sounded lifeless and agitatedly monotone to himself, as if he wanted to be alone.

The walk began to seem flickeringly, harshly, unsteadily surreal. Tao focused on asking questions. He learned Finn and Paetra had been in a relationship for four years, that she was the "most wholesome" woman he'd dated, that he'd dated intravenous heroin users, and that Kathleen had fallen through a second-floor stairwell in Mexico in 2008 and been badly injured. Finn, who lived in Santa Rosa with a roommate, prefaced the last with something like "I don't know if she told you or not but" and Tao said she hadn't. Finn said he'd lived in the house for one and a half years after the accident, taking care of his mom, the house, and the garden.

Tao had anticipated it since June 16, when Kathleen said, "Occidental hosts a charming and lively farmers market each Friday, 4pm to dark, which is kind of a street party with music and beautiful vegetables" in an email, and now the market's peacefully bustling ambience and varied offerings dissolved the walk's relatively foreboding mood. It was on a fragment of street beginning and ending in Occidental and had at least twenty-eight stands, including ones selling fermented beverages and vegetables, non-factory-farmed meat, organic gluten-free spring rolls, made-to-order smoothies, baskets of greens, tiny plums, and face painting. Relative to the size of Occidental, the market was around equivalent to, Tao later estimated using Google Earth, Manhattan hosting a market filling Central Park.

That night, Tao went outside twice to walk, jog, and breathe. He felt better after each brief trip—calmer, stabler, less neurotic, less gloomy. In five months, in December, the *Journal of Neuroscience* would publish a paper on how people recognized fearful faces faster and had better short-term memory when inhaling than exhaling, but only when inhaling through the nose. "When you breathe in, we discovered you are stimulating neurons in the olfactory cortex, amygdala and hippocampus," said Christina Zelano, the lead author of the paper, which would remind Tao of the hours and days in his childhood and as an adult when his nose, due to various twentieth-century reasons, had been completely obstructed with mucous and/or sometimes dried blood; reading the paper, he'd consider how contemporary children, being more toxified and degenerate and immobile and inflamed than he'd been in the 1980s and 1990s, must be mouthbreathing even more than he had as a child. He was probably stronger now than he'd ever been, which he suspected contributed to his breaking his computer. Parts of him probably hadn't realized his body moved less weakly and tentatively now.

Two nights earlier—before returning to San Remo Hotel and cracking his computer's screen—he'd also enjoyed moving around outside. He'd walked, sat, lay, jogged, ran, stretched, and breathed in Fort Mason Park for around two hours, the Golden Gate Bridge small and fog-framed in the distance. On the low-lit, hilly sidewalks of North Beach, he'd skipped in three rhythms, skipping more than he had since some forgotten day in childhood. Society associated skipping with children and viewed it, a fractal form of walking, jogging, and running, as feminine. Tao wanted to do it more. His shoes had 3-millimeter soles. In the past, he'd worn shoes that separated him from the ground by 25.4 to 63.5 mm or 1 to 2.5 inches. Like most people, he'd turned his feet into densely mitted, awkwardly club-like things, treating them as if they were severely injured and required thick casts. Tao had learned this "cast" metaphor from *Move Your DNA* (2014) by Katy Bowman, who also applied it to vision, observing that rooms were like casts on the muscles in our eyes that changed the shape of our lens so we could focus different distances.

Tao could move only four of his ten toes. Staring at five toes, he was unable to mentally focus in a manner causing the middle three to individually move, but, partly because sometimes one or two would twiddle a little, he sensed the skill existed. He'd never noticed this inability until recently, and it had seemed strange and interesting. For the first time, he'd sensed a physical inability as a kind of deadness. Six of his toes seemed numb and uncontrollable from disuse. He imagined that parts of the deforested, razed, replaced wilderness of his mind—filled with tens of thousands of hours of TV, video and computer games, public education, pornography, mass media, movies, literary fiction, nightmares, and dreams—must also be partially to fully nonfunctioning, that probably there were mental abilities he'd forgotten or never learned, ones he could discover, revive, nourish, and use.

As Tao's interest in nature, psychedelics, the possibility that life ended with a release into a higher-dimensional place called the imagination, and his mind increased, so did his interest in microbes, his body, nutrition, and other physical topics. By self-consciously, note-takingly exercising and stretching in a variety of physical and mental states in the past three years, including in Taipei doing yoga in a class alternating days of baked cannabis and 50 to 100 micrograms of LSD, he'd learned that he often unconsciously held some of his muscles, especially in his neck and jaws and shoulders and back, in sustained tension and that, in this way, his unconscious seemed to have a kind of control over his body. He'd theorized that he was unable, as a twenty-first-century degenerate, to generate enough consciousness to be aware of his entire body and surroundings and mind at one time; therefore he sometimes seemed to become aware of his muscles having been "unconsciously tensed" for unknown amounts of time.

After his two brief walks/jogs, Tao emailed his mom saying

he was happy her mouth pain was "not something serious." He told her about the market and said people in Occidental seemed healthy, that he "ate many organic blueberries and bought organic fermented cabbage and a fermented turmeric drink," and that the plant-drawing class was the next day from 10:00 A.M. to 4:00 P.M. Tao had learned the term "organic," which in Taiwan was 有機 (yŏujī), in college, maybe in 2003, while researching how to feel less depressed, tired, and anxious. Once, in San Francisco in 2010, on book tour, he'd overheard a new friend criticizing "organic" as a marketing scam; he'd told the friend that organically certified food was grown without synthetic pesticides, among other restrictions. "Oh, then that means something, then," the friend had said earnestly, having believed, probably due to being naturally suspicious of adjectives applied to products, the term was a meaningless abstraction like "best" or "high-quality."

Before sleep, Tao thought about how that day he'd maybe embodied the role of a normal person too much and too often. In the garden, he'd said his book was secondary, that he was just a normal person taking a drawing class, doing what he wanted to do in life. In the moment, he'd overstated his position, he now felt, and then had begun to act that way. To idly sit there, patiently enjoying the situation—as if for some reason pretending he wasn't going to write about any of this—instead of remaining inquisitive, extra-alert, and time-sensitively exploratory.

The next day, Tao told himself, he would be more journalistic. He liked being journalistic—focusing on others with heightened attention, noticing details and behaviors, asking series of questions. He'd called his book secondary, but sometimes he preferred viewing his life as secondary and his books and other writing—the selective downloads of his life—as primary. Since college, when he began creating linguistic, sharable, fractal microcosms of his life in the form of short stories and poems, experience and literature had become increasingly symbiotic for him—a trend that made him curious about the future.

3. THE PLANT-DRAWING CLASS

Kathleen introduced herself, the class, and her former student Paetra, who said a little about herself, and then the students began to introduce themselves. After a few introductions, Tao remembered his plan to be more journalistic—toward others but also toward the higher-dimensional character of himself, who seemed to become more controllable the more he recovered— and began recording a Voice Memo with his phone on his chair by his thighs. Holding up his arm and turning it self-consciously in various directions, feeling a little nervous, Tao said he lived in New York City and used to draw simple things, like the red hamster tattoo on his hand, but was now drawing more complex things and had recently noticed nature made complex things, which made this class perfect for him. A woman in her fifties said she'd been zooming into plants and drawing them at up to 600× magnification. Finn, seated in back, said he found his mom's classes "fascinating, psychologically." He alluded to "long psychoanalytical sessions" that happened afterward with his mom and maybe others. Tao imagined them analyzing human behavior and felt interested. A bearded man in his twenties with glasses had traveled there from Oregon. A man named Daniel had sold Tao plums the day before at the farmers market. Around half the students in the filled, fifteen-student class cited Kathleen and her work as a reason they were there, and around half had attended a previous BD event.

Tao sat opposite Corinne, adjacent Frances, and diagonal

Emelia. Corinne was in her sixties and wryly and endearingly self-critical. Frances was shy and taciturn and smiley and had a nose ring and was dressed like a punk. Emelia, the youngest student, was in high school; her presence gave the room, day, and class a slightly futuristic quality. Tao felt excited for her and imagined others also vicariously feeling what she felt, or what they imagined she felt, as a teenager in a non-school-related, somewhat obscure plant-drawing class on a Saturday morning in July 2016. Tao was amused to hear Emelia, at one point, meekly say, "Hm?" to Corinne, who responded, "Oh, nothing, I was just talking to myself."

As Kathleen demonstrated tools while speaking on and around the topic of botanical illustration in a range of tones, regularly eliciting laughter, her fingers sometimes shimmered or blurred or vibrated in non-physical ways, it seemed to Tao, who was the kind of stoned where concrete reality felt slightly ajar and light from elsewhere seemed almost able to get through, making things seem realer and more captivating from obscurely increased dimensionality. Kathleen reminded the students to breathe and Tao realized he'd been breathing shallowly—as he had most of his life—and began taking deep, long breaths, looking around a little. He'd read an email that morning from his mom that said, "Another 2.5 hours, 5:02 is the time you were born 33 years ago. Here I wish you the best, healthiest and happiest birthday ever."

As students moved in and out of the library—deciding what to draw, gathering tools—Tao located Finn and began praising his family's garden. He said he regretted not exploring and photographing and tasting it more the day before. Finn said he was welcome to visit again. Tao said he was leaving that night, though. "And so a second garden visit remained uncertain," he thought while returning to his seat to focus on drawing the ginkgo leaf he'd picked that morning by Bohemian Highway, at the entrance to Harmony Village. He'd been surprised to see the lone, flame-shaped ginkgo tree there.

Later, around ten minutes after stopping the Voice Memo, Tao began recording a second Voice Memo, found a semi-busy-seeming Finn, and asked him how many species of plants were in his family's garden. Finn said he didn't know. Hadn't counted. He was gathering drawing tools and seemed a bit distracted. Tao asked if he could estimate at all. To his amusement and approval, Finn then seemed to move away, back toward his seat, in a manner one might depart someone asking annoying questions. Tao imagined Finn being quietly brusque with him from then on—as people should be with overbearing journalists, he thought while grinning to himself.

A little later, Tao found himself outside with Finn by the table of plant parts to potentially draw. He felt stoned and caffeinated to a degree that he felt friendly and playful with almost everyone. Suddenly and with awkward language, he asked Finn how many greens the garden had that could be eaten in a salad.

"You're really into this quantitative thing, aren't you?"

Tao laughed. His best question as a journalist, the first he'd asked that day, had been how many species were in the garden. Now his second question was also focused on how many of something existed. Tao considered explicating a little (he wanted to use numbers to gain a more accurate sense of the relative diversity and size and scale of things) or defending himself (the question was deliberately awkward and objective so his subject could feel comfortable and helpful at the beginning of an interaction, which might lead elsewhere) but then focused, instead, on Finn, who was naming species from the Brassicaceae family, of which the garden had many, including kale, mustard, and arugula.

After that, Tao felt he'd behaved journalistically enough for the day and stopped recording. He'd created five Voice Memos, which seemed like enough. If he visited the garden again, he would be journalistic there—in an unforced and limited way, photographing and listening and noting—but otherwise he'd try to be his normal, nonbelligerent self. He'd gone too far, maybe, after the affirmation the night before, in the journalistic direction; or maybe, he suggested to himself, he'd gone just far enough, creating an overall, commensal balance, reporting-wise, between the temporal dyad of the day before and that day.

During the lunch break, students and teachers sat in sunlight in the middle of Harmony Village. It took the sun 226 million years to orbit the black hole at the center of their galaxy, whose diameter was 0.15 million light-years. Light from their galaxy took 2.54 million years to reach Andromeda, the nearest non-satellite galaxy. In four to five billion years, the two galaxies, which together had at least 1.1 trillion stars and were each orbited by tens of satellite galaxies, would collide, becoming one. Tao felt friendly and even garrulous, peaking on a capsule of coconut oil, turmeric powder, black pepper, and 0.3 grams of cannabis—a plant he was still learning how to use after three years of constant, varied alliance. He met Klea and her daughter, Fiona, who seemed uncannily discerning, like she was 102, not almost 2. Feeling slightly surreal as he behaved with uncharacteristic charisma, Tao found himself "openly hinting," he felt, that he'd like to see the garden again. Kathleen said he could visit the garden after class since he'd already been there once and had come all the way from New

York. Tao realized some students—three or four within earshot—might be wondering why he was allowed to see Kathleen's garden after class. He hadn't told anyone he was a writer.

"Do you think you want to have children?" he asked Finn.

Finn repeated Tao's question, then they and others laughed.

Finn said he would. He would like to have children.

A student named Chris said California's Central Valley was full of pesticides, attracting Tao's attention. Pesticides, Tao knew, had been invented during World War II for use in chemical warfare and to kill insects, then corporations had sold them to people and governments for use in killing rodents, birds, insects, plants, fungi, microorganisms, and other life-forms. As modern people spread pesticides across the planet in the 1950s and 1960s, aboriginals had spread psychedelics (psilocybin, salvia, ayahuasca) to modern people, and then both pesticides and psychedelics had spread, from the 1960s to the 2010s, into bodies and cities, fields and brains, food products and drug stashes. Chris and Tao discussed smog. Tao had read a Swedish paper recently that linked mental illness in children with air pollution. Eating avocado and fermented cabbage, Tao said he wanted to move to Santa Cruz.

Another student, named Ellie, also had a glass jar of fermented vegetables, he'd noticed. Every aboriginal and "traditional"—a differentiation on the aboriginal-modern spectrum—society that Weston A. Price visited in the 1930s preserved and nutritionally enriched their food via fermentation, which transformed food into stable homes for beneficial microbes, Tao knew from *Wild Fermentation* (2003) and other books. Tens of trillions of bacteria, fungi, archaea, and protists, representing probably one to five hundred species, lived in his eyes, mouth, esophagus, stomach, intestines, genitals, skin, and lungs. Each microbe was a cell made of up to tens of millions of giant molecules called proteins. Each microbe affected Tao's consciousness at all times by, among other means, creating neurotransmitters and other compounds for him to absorb, including ones he needed but couldn't make, like vitamins C, K2, B1, B2, B5, B6, B7, B9, and B12.

Pesticides—different types of which killed different microbes—were one reason why the three to four generations of people born since World War II had significantly less diverse, helpful, and stable microbiotas than their thousands of generations of ancestors. In *Silent Spring*, marine biologist Rachel Carson (1907–1964) wrote that pesticides, which she viewed as a major threat to human existence, had been underestimated as a problem because, among other reasons, they caused damage that was "almost impossible to trace to its origins." Carson had breast cancer when *Silent Spring* was published in September 1962—after being serialized that summer in the *New Yorker*—and died nineteen months later of a heart attack. Due in part to her book, her fourth after three on the sea, the Environmental Protection Agency was created in 1970 and some pesticides were eventually banned—DDT in 1972, aldrin in 1974, heptachlor in 1978—but these and other compounds, plus their metabolites, like DDD and DDE, were still, in 2015, detectable in food due to their "persistence in the environment," according to the U.S. Department of Agriculture's annual Pesticide Data Program report.

Banning those and other pesticides meant relatively little, Tao had learned, because hundreds of others, in the meantime, since the 1970s, had been invented, marketed, sold, and heavily used. In its 2015 PDP report, the USDA explained it had tested 10,187 samples of food (360 certified organic) for 465 pesticides, metabolites, degradates, and isomers and that, after washing and blending the samples, 14 types of pesticides had been found in lettuce, 16 in apples and peaches, 20 in cherries and pears, 23 in spinach, 27 in tomatoes, and 38 in strawberries, to name some common foods, even though they didn't test for all pesticides.

One pesticide not tested for was glyphosate, which Monsanto began selling in 1974 in its product Roundup for killing plants. Seven hundred tons of glyphosate were used globally that year, 73,941 tons in 1995, and 910,292 tons in 2014, when the United States, with 4.5 percent of the planet's population, used 15 percent of the glyphosate, which killed by, among many other ways, disabling an enzyme used by plants, fungi, and microbes to create the aromatic amino acids, including two that animals required but did not make—phenylalanine (used by turmeric to make curcuminoids, plants to make vitamin E, and animals to make opioids and dopamine) and tryptophan, which some fungi used to make psilocybin and animals used to make serotonin and DMT and other compounds.

Meaning that because of the one pesticide glyphosate, which was in air, soil, rain, surface and ground water, tap water, non-organic cotton and tobacco and food, and vaccines in amounts confirmed or suspected, due to increasing usage, to be rising over time, most or potentially all twenty-first-century humans were deficient, to some degree, in at least three amino acids, nine vitamins, twenty opioids including six endorphins, dopamine, adrenaline (made from dopamine), serotonin, melatonin (made from serotonin), and DMT.

During Tao's childhood in Florida, in the 1980s and 1990s, seemingly every family had used an array of synthetic poisons in and on their homes, vehicles, lawns, and pets—"bug sprays" and "weed killers" and cockroach traps and flea collars and other essential-seeming products that civilized, sedentary people had existed without for more than ten thousand years. Parks, businesses, schools, and houses had been fumigated regularly. The familiar, woozy, deadly scent had seemed unharmful and even vaguely comforting. When, at age eighteen, Tao left for New York City, the city of him probably contained parts per million or billion of glyphosate—which had been in vaccines since probably the late seventies because vaccines contained soy, sucrose, and various proteins from non-organic sources and because some viruses, like measles, shingles, and flu, were grown on gelatin derived from pigs and cows fed genetically modified food containing up to 400 parts per million of the 18-atom compound, which Tao would eventually think of as "the bleakest drug"—plus hundreds to thousands of other synthetic compounds, making him malfunction socially, physically, cognitively, psychologically, and emotionally in obvious, subtle, subconscious, layered, and unpredictable ways.

Tao used to think of his body as a small, swamp-like thing, where anything could be tossed without concern because it'd disappear into the overall stew of him. Encouraged by corporations and governmental organizations and media that parroted those sources, which said there were "safe" levels of compounds that had been introduced decades earlier to biological systems that had evolved without them for billions of years, he felt he could throw things into the pile of his body and they would dissolve, or something. Now he viewed his body as an enormous city in which each molecule of BPA, PVC, PCB, and CFC, of ethylmercury and phthalate and polyethylene and anti-depressant, flame retardant and surfactant and artificial sweetener, neonicotinoid and organophosphate, was a nonfunctioning, havoc-causing member of society—that would not be absorbed into the murky bog of him and be forgotten but would have a concrete effect on the molecular city of him during its life-span as itself and multiple metabolites. There was no "safe" level, it now seemed to Tao; the effects began, on him and his microbe symbionts, at one molecule and increased from there and also varied by person.

Silent Spring, which Tao read in February, a week and a half before starting his book, memorably contributed to his reconceptualization. In one passage, Carson wrote that scientists had found the food of Eskimos to be DDT-free except for two migratory owls, but that some Eskimos themselves, in 1961, contained up to 1.9 ppm of DDT, which Monsanto and other corporations began selling in 1944, because they'd undergone surgery in a hospital in Anchorage. "For their brief stay in civilization the Eskimos were rewarded with a taint of poison," wrote Carson, who observed that, because DDT was stored in fat, an intake of 0.1 ppm could be magnified in storage to 10 to 15 ppm, which the body would experience when it used its fat reserves, at which point the effects would most likely be obliviously misattributed. "One part in a million sounds like a very small amount—and so it is," wrote Carson about the 28-atom, colorless, tasteless compound. "But such substances are so potent that a minute quantity can bring about vast changes in the body." In animal experiments, 5 ppm of DDT and 2.5 ppm of the also-common pesticides dieldrin and chlordane, banned in 1974 and 1988, killed liver cells.

Those findings—and other evidence that twenty-first-century humans were deeply unoptimized—meant to Tao that there was a lot of potential for life to feel less arduous and nauseating, more satisfying and enchanting, than it had so far. Due to malnutrition, pesticides, the overuse of synthetic antibiotics (a twentieth-century invention that, like pesticides, harmed in difficult-to-trace ways, like by altering the human microbiome over generations cumulatively), and other problems, like air pollution and plastic contamination and hundreds of nuclear power plants continually producing radioactive waste, humans in 2016 did not feel like humans 100,000, 10,000, 100, or even 10 years ago. Because diet, environment, and microbiota are the main factors determining the ingredients of the drug cocktail of the drug trip of life, humans felt different than ever before.

When Tao encountered Terence in 2012, he'd initially been most intrigued and excited by his theory that humans were near the chaotic end of a dimension-rending transformation called history—and that the task, then, was to remain calm and do something to facilitate the birth-like, unnatural-seeming, difficult, delicate, failable process. Humans couldn't return to grassland nomadism or even the nineteenth century, but if we survived long enough we might leave Earth behind, like a placenta, in a "forward escape" into the imagination. The theory had seemed startling and convincing—systems in the universe did seem to naturally complexify at an accelerating rate, from cells to animals to Çatalhöyük to New York City to the internet—and, with its attached suggestion of helping instead of panicking or freezing in worry and anxiety, it continued to influence Tao and to attract his investigative attention.

The end of history, he was now gradually learning, was feelable. It felt like being unwittingly poisoned, like something was pervasively wrong. The younger one was, the more one felt it, but it was a feeling everyone alive, near the end of time, closely shared, apparently. Tao was glad to be continuing to learn and increasingly understand all this. That he'd felt bad as a child and adult not for "no concrete reason" but for reasons so tiny they were nearly invisible. And now also for invisible—electromagnetic—reasons, which he'd learned about from *An Electronic Silent Spring* (2014), which described the carcinogenic and other effects of radiation from wireless technology, computers, smart meters, microwave ovens, and smartphones.

———

Back in class, Tao checked on Finn, who was drawing a poppy pod, then sat and focused on his ginkgo leaf. Kathleen had said if students showed detail in selected areas, the viewer would fill in the rest. Tao was attracted to this selection-based technique, but his leaf seemed so small and simple—most students had chosen multi-parted subjects—that it seemed joke-like to only detail some of it. After hearing Corinne talk to herself about wanting to abandon her drawing—which seemed, to her, bad—Tao said he also wanted to start over and then was surprised when Corinne strongly encouraged him to keep going. Minutes later, he quietly started over on the back of his paper. Corinne had been bluffing about wanting to start over, he thought with a mental grin.

Kathleen sometimes inflected the class with a relationship metaphor, pointing out the at-some-point-necessary decision to "commit" to one's drawing, referencing the choice of whether one wanted to sleep with one's drawing. Tao heard her tell a student that fractals were hard to draw and remembered he'd recently written "Fractals are difficult to draw" in his book. He was struggling, he felt, with his ginkgo leaf. Kathleen photographed it with her phone and minutes later returned with a zoomed-in, X-ray-looking image of the leaf with every part, it seemed, visible.

After redrawing it and feeling unsatisfied like before, Tao began to feel the stimulating and jostling effects of a cannabis capsule he used after lunch (his second capsule of the day) and privately acknowledged he was trying to draw something related to his book—two weeks earlier, he'd noticed *Ginkgo biloba* in Washington Square Park for the first time and since then had been surprised to find the plant, which he'd written into his book's chapter on cannabis, wherever in Manhattan he went—and was forcing it and it wasn't working. Finally letting his plans evolve, he began drawing a pin oak leaf he'd also picked that morning.

Near the end of class, Tao said his computer was broken and asked Kathleen if she had a charger for his phone. Kathleen asked if his computer broke while "here." Thinking of California, Tao answered, somewhat vaguely, "yes." Speaking partially then to around four people, Tao said he'd broken his computer by accident while trying to fix it, then thanked Kathleen and returned to his seat. Kathleen had taught the class how to further dimensionalize drawings by indicating a light source, and now Tao applied the technique to his twenty-nine-tip pin oak leaf, which he'd quickly sketched down, in one area, to the smallest visible shapes outlined by the reticulating subveins, impressing himself.

At the end of class, teachers temporarily framed and showed each drawing and said descriptive, analytical, encouraging comments. Students also commented. Sometimes there were discussions, digressions, and sub-discussions, including one on the possible synergistic effects of opium poppy and carrot greens, which Chris had drawn as a pair. Paetra, discussing three or four pieces, pointed out plants' whimsical and comical aspects. Kathleen directed attention toward plants' aesthetics. She indicated the specific leaf in a black-and-white drawing that to her conveyed the plant was silvery. "It reminds me of Botanical Dimensions's logo," said Tao at the end of the discussion on Corinne's drawing, which students and teachers felt exuded an offbeat, restrained humor while also seeming somewhat wild and even bursting.

Immediately after class, Tao walked quickly to Union Hotel—because he wanted to stay another night and Occidental Hotel had no vacancies—and learned it wasn't a hotel. It was an Italian restaurant (Occidental had two), a general store, a bar, and, it seemed, one or two other establishments. Tao felt like he was on a cruise ship. He found his way outside and walked for around a minute in pleasurably warm sunlight to Inn at Occidental, which he learned was expensive—for marriages and honeymoons, it seemed. He wouldn't stay another night, then.

Part of what he was experiencing, as an animal, was his feelings, a large part of which came from the ever-changing statuses, quantity, distribution, and level of functioning of his neurotransmitter receptors, of which he had at least 141 types, including nineteen purinergic, fourteen serotonergic, eleven adrenergic, nine opioid, five dopaminergic, and probably three cannabinoid. His feelings existed with what his other receptors, like ones for vision and olfaction and other senses, detected. As an anatomically modern human, he also had language, with which he continually influenced his feelings from a metaphysical direction. He had the opportunity to experience emotions at this gradation of subtlety and level of control and awareness—a gift of complexity that could be overwhelming to almost unbearable, sometimes making him cry from appreciation and incredulity and confusion—because billions of his ancestors' siblings had died young, leaving more resources for the survivors: his ancestors.

Each of Tao's billions of ancestors, going back to shrews and fish and earlier, had been strong and motivated enough to survive and reproduce—consecutively, over billions of years, through five mass extinctions and thousands of global cataclysms, in an incredible living streak, never starving or being eaten or succumbing to shyness or accident or religion, or some other temperament or circumstance or interest, before reproducing. Tao's parents had survived and passed on their DNA, and so had their parents, and so on. Billions of moms and dads had survived. Tao felt especially impressed by this reality—the improbability of which he'd only recently begun to realize—because he felt he could have easily died already and because he felt he could easily live the rest of his life without reproducing, thus casually ending the streak.

Walking back to the library, at the T-shaped intersection with the ginkgo tree, Tao saw Klea and Fiona across the street. He and Klea waved and then there was a moderately loud rumbling in the near distance. Facing the noise with her upper body, as if on guard, Fiona cowered cutely in a different direction toward her mom. "Oh, that's just a motorcycle," said Klea.

Outside the library, Finn told Tao they thought he'd left. And that he'd left his phone. Tao said he hadn't left, that he was excited to be in the garden again. Corinne and Chris and other students were helping move things and tidy the library—of their own volition, Tao knew, as Kathleen had explicitly said not to worry about it. Students seemed reluctant to leave. Tao smiled and waved bye to a smiling, leaving Frances—who'd drawn the most impressive, people had seemed to agree, piece—and entered the library.

"What's your birthday?" said Paetra to him suddenly. Taken aback, in part because he'd decided with satisfaction to just not mention his birthday, Tao asked why. Paetra said she did astrology. Tao said his birthday was that day. Paetra observed, then Tao confirmed, that he was taking a plant-drawing class on his birthday. Paetra then Kathleen hugged him.

"You're thirty-three?" said Finn, and Tao, feeling amused (slightly now and more later in contemplation) that Finn, who'd also homed in on age when introducing his thirty-five-year-old friend, focused on the topic's main quantitative aspect, said he was.

Outside, on the sidewalk, minutes later, Tao heard Paetra and Finn talking about Finn's headache, which he'd had for hours and for which he'd used an Advil. Tao sympathetically discussed headaches with Finn while moving things to his car.

By the car, Finn and Tao assessed the class. It had gone

well. Finn said people had sometimes come to Terence's talks on drugs—someone would begin dancing, someone on mushrooms. He said Kathleen hadn't attracted anyone like that.

"Someone get this boy a birthday cake!" shouted Paetra as she drove away.

Kathleen told Chris, who'd driven from Berkeley and had attended other BD events, they were going to her garden and that he was welcome to join.

Getting into Kathleen's car, Tao thought he'd lost his phone then found it after seconds. "It was in my pocket," he said to Kathleen. "I found it," he said across the parking lot to Finn, who was riding with Chris. "It was in my pocket."

Driving to her house, Kathleen said she felt really good after planning, creating, promoting, preparing, and teaching the class. She seemed energized and ready to teach another class. In the passenger seat, Tao briefly felt he should be interviewing her like a TV reporter might with an athlete who'd just won something. He said it was good to bring like-minded people together.

Kathleen said Paetra, who'd been her student at the California School of Herbal Studies, once was going to marry a South American man. Kathleen was going to officiate the wedding. But then the wedding had been canceled. Then Kathleen had thought, "Finn would like Paetra," and now, after a four-year relationship that ended six years earlier, the two were best friends. Kathleen said she'd been set to officiate nonoccurring weddings twice in her life.

Tao said he'd noticed Finn and Paetra had a playful, witty rapport that seemed fun and intimate. Tao himself had been married since 2010, when he was twenty-seven. He and his wife, Megan, had separated in 2011, but they'd procrastinated since then on getting a divorce, which would cost hundreds of dollars and require many forms and a number of notary public, court, and post office visits. Like Finn and Paetra, they'd remained friends, though they lived in different states and communicated intermittently.

At Kathleen's house, Tao opened his door through his open window, eliciting congratulations on learning. Exiting the car, he heard Kathleen tell Klea, who was standing in the driveway, he'd gotten too stoned the day before and had forgotten to take pictures and videos and explore the garden, so was back to do those things now. He asked Finn how he'd describe the house's shape.

"Wedge-shaped. Terence used to call it 'the wedge at the edge.'"

Tao asked if he could photograph it and Finn said yes.

Walking toward it after photographing it, Tao noticed the house, which he'd two-dimensionally thought of as a "triangle" because he'd first seen the polyhedron triangle-side-on and because he didn't know the name "right triangular prism" or think of the word "wedge," had a second, baby wedge, connected at its top to the main wedge's bottom. The others sat by the shed and Tao explored the garden alone, touching and smelling and eating new and familiar plants. In a week, back in the city, where the trees grew away from the buildings for sunlight and probably other reasons, he would read Kathleen's essay on tripping in nature, "Treat Her Right: Lessons from a Medicine Walk" (2009), which began "To begin with, I'll go out on a limb: Nature loves it when we take psychedelics and wander around, appreciating her, in a state of respectful awe and gratitude." In the five-part essay, which included a first-person-plural nature walk and a part on the use of psychedelics by activists, artists, and scientists, he would read: "I think one of the coolest causes is bringing very urban kids to the country, the forest, or the shore, the kind of places they've never seen." He would read:

> Be careful, I must warn you, watch your step! The plants and fungi have been known to hijack humans! Many of us! Of course, those of us who've been hijacked seem to be pretty darn happy about it, so there's that. But so many people have turned toward plants, toward growing things, from what they thought was their career, it's laughable.

Tao sat and smoked cannabis with Kathleen, Finn, and Chris. He wandered back into the garden once or twice to breathe and eat more plants. He ate a seven-leaflet cannabis leaf, finding it surprisingly nutty. When Finn handed him the pipe a second or third time, he acknowledged and felt excited at the possibility— low, he felt, but not zero—that Finn had for some reason spiked it with something. Kathleen, who'd abstained the day before, smoked that day. Cannabis was probably significantly stronger for her, Tao considered with vicarious excitement, than for him, who since February had begun smoking within an hour of waking most days and continued into the night, though not uncontrollably but around 0.6 g per day. Besides "sober," life for Kathleen had at least two other distinct, historied, familiar settings (caffeine, which interacted with her adenosine and glycine and other receptors, and cannabis), usefully triangulating her daily experience and, among other effects, stabilizing her, Tao imagined.

In four months, in November, Nevada, Massachusetts, Maine, and California would relegalize cannabis, and six months after that, Tao would develop a Kathleen-inspired method of not smoking until five hours after waking. Two months after that, in July 2017, while finishing the fifth and final draft of his book, Tao would learn that twenty-first-century humans were even less stoned and more inflamed than he'd so far realized; that month, a paper would announce the discovery that mammals convert DHEA and EPEA—endocannabinoids created from DHA and EPA, which are found mostly in animal fats—into more potent, previously unknown endocannabinoids that interacted with both CB1 and CB2 receptors and had "enhanced anti-inflammatory properties." The conversion was made by CYP enzymes, which, Tao would know from a 2013 paper by Anthony Samsel and Stephanie Seneff, were suppressed by glyphosate.

Kathleen led Tao and Chris, who was six-five or six-six and affably bearish, on a smell and taste tour of her garden. Tao made a six-second video of a species of *Digitales* that was taller than him. Its flowers looked like painted models of tunnels with little entities rushing out or being suctioned in—only on the bottom, making the colored dots seem affected by gravity.

"Do you have a—garden at all?" said Kathleen in the video.

"Not so much," said Chris. "I have a couple of houseplants."

Tao said his room had no direct sunlight or plants. For around 10,700 generations, from 280,000 to 12,000 years ago, the diets of his ancestors had probably averaged much more than a hundred plant species, each with its own distinct configuration of common, uncommon, rare, and unique compounds. The Sierra Miwok, for example, who once lived in central California, used around 160 species for food and 110 for medicine, suffusing themselves in minerals, amino acids, phytoncides, antioxidants, anti-inflammatants, neurotransmitters, polyphenols, terpenes, anthocyanins, carotenoids, chlorophylls, vitamins, peptides, enzymes, and other phytocompounds. Humans began eating fewer plant species when they condensed into permanent settlements—at Çatalhöyük, 8,000 years or 320 generations ago,

fourteen food species were grown and others were foraged—
but still more, and more nourishingly, than in the twentieth and
twenty-first centuries, when most people, genetically starved for
nutrition from microbes, fungi, insects, animals, and plants,
were suffused in compounds that had been invented less than
five generations ago and were sold not with hundreds of others in
the nutritious matrix of a leaf, seed, root, rhizome, bulb, or fruit
but with ten or so other toxic ingredients in the surreally crude
dead zones of pills, tablets, creams, pastes, sunscreens, and processed foods.

They looked at a three-dimensional spider web that seemed
absurdly and extravagantly complex—a mansion with thousands
of rooms, each a different size, fitting in every direction. There
was something comical about the level of complexity, but instead
of laughing, Tao felt himself become more attentive.

Eyes closed, he chewed what he thought was lemon balm,
which Finn, from a distance, had recommended they taste. Kathleen asked what he saw and Tao said the star from Super Mario
Bros. He explained that, in the video game, one jumped on things
to kill them but with the star you could run through them.

He learned he'd chewed catnip, not lemon balm, then said
that "lemon balm" had maybe influenced what he saw because
"lemon" had made him think yellow—the color of the star item.

Finn joined the tour and Tao looked at a hazelnut wrapped in
an octopus-costume-like covering that was a lighter green than
the kelpy, rippling leaves it seemed to float among.

After smelling a species with three colors of flower, each with
a different scent, they approached what Tao thought of as Raspberry Fortress, which seemed like a magically blown-up, living,
plant version of the spider's web-complex.

Tao showed Finn a tiny raspberry and said it was cute and
Finn grinned and agreed. Tao pulled a raspberry and it slid off,

revealing a white, stalagmite-ish cone. He recorded his left hand removing a raspberry and thought, "Decapping the stalagmite."

Kathleen brought him a peppery orange flower, which he ate.

Finn encouraged Chris and Tao to eat a tomato leaf and they did.

Kathleen went inside to get travel information for Tao. She returned and told Chris the plan: Drive Tao to Cotati. As Tao and Chris left the garden, Finn jogged to them, offering blueberries from his palm. Tao overheard that Klea was going to cook dinner for Fiona, Finn, and her mom. On the driveway, he noticed a front-yard area that was steeply sloped and bonsai-like, covered with a rococo verdure of plants. He began to think of the property as a garden containing a house, cottage, shed, and driveway.

By Chris's car, Finn felt peaches—less rapidly than his mom but with a similarly "peacefully frenzied," Tao felt, way of maneuvering the branches—while talking and chose three or four and gave Tao one, which Tao ate, then another, which Tao put in his bag. Tao confirmed he had enough cannabis for later, then said bye to Kathleen and her children, thanking them.

Four weeks later, he would decide what to mail them as a thank-you gift—*Nourishing Traditions* (1995), a 688-page cookbook based on the findings of Weston A. Price that began with an essay with 188 scientific references supporting the wisdom of aboriginals on food and health. "Technology can be a kind father but only in partnership with his mothering, feminine partner—the nourishing traditions of our ancestors," wrote Sally Fallon in the preface to her cookbook, which Tao would mail with a typed letter that began "I've been writing with pleasure about my trip."

On the 8:15 P.M. bus from Cotati to San Francisco, Tao handwrote memories of the unrecorded parts of his day in the notebook he'd bought hours before breaking his computer, then on yelp.com found a hotel with an average rating of four stars, shared bathrooms, and, according to one review, "EXTREMELY thin" walls. It was called Union Hotel, like the non-hotel establishment in Occidental. Tao called and reserved a room, then emailed his mom, saying he was on a bus, and in the email attached a photo of the wedge-shaped house.

4. SAN FRANCISCO

After disembarking at 5th Street, Tao walked south on Mission Street, smoking cannabis from a glass one-hitter he'd bought around there three days earlier, in transit from SFO to San Remo Hotel. He noticed the taco place he ate at with the ska/punk man after his reading in Petaluma seven years earlier. He ordered takeout of half a roasted chicken from a bar/restaurant on Valencia, then walked south to 21st Street, remembering times he'd been here and sometimes, while feeling lucid and alert, calmly forgetting where he was—in which city and when, as whom.

In Union Hotel, on Mission and 16th, around 11:15 P.M., Tao texted a photo of his gray-blue bed to his mom, calling it cozy and cute. The hotel, which seemed to be operated by three generations of an Indian family living behind the main counter, smelled strongly of cumin, clove, paprika, dill, cinnamon, nutmeg, fennel, chili pepper, star anise, and other Indian-food spices, to Tao's approval and delighted satisfaction. His aversion to artificial scents had increased significantly in the past few years. He ate chicken and turmeric sauerkraut and drank mineral water. Writing memories in his notebook, he felt densely, pleasurably stoned.

That night, he woke to sex from two heterosexual couples— first one, later another—that seemed loud enough for everyone on the floor, maybe in the hotel, to hear. Tao hadn't had sex, or even kissed anyone, in almost three years, which didn't feel especially aberrant to him—even though since 2002 he'd been in five relationships each lasting around a year—because he'd had other periods in his life, like ages one to nineteen and when he was twenty-one and twenty-two, among other ages, when, with varying amounts of loneliness, he'd refrained, by choice and/or not, from romantic and sexual relationships, focusing instead, in ways that sometimes encouragingly reminded him of being a child happily playing alone, on other things.

Like with DMT in 2012, 2013, and 2014, Tao felt he should "recover more" before trying relationships beyond friendship. Having hermit-like tendencies, a job and main interest in life that was solitary, and generally liking being alone, celibacy hadn't been difficult for him. Someday, he'd try romantic and sexual relationships again, or maybe he wouldn't. He could just focus on all these other things now. The more he learned, the more alienated he felt from others and the harder it became to find people with similar perspectives. Which was another reason for his book. So people could know what he knew. So he wouldn't feel alone in knowing.

Another reason—the fifth—for his book was that he wanted to learn the ideas, stories, discoveries, reconceptualizations, statistics, and other information that he'd put in it. Without the book, he wouldn't have learned its content as fast or maybe ever. He wouldn't have sought, read, reread, created, contemplated, and experimented with phrases, sentences, paragraphs, parts, and chapters about the topics in it six to thirteen hours a day, around 97 percent of days, for seventeen months. His book was an effect of teaching himself its content. After it was published, he would occasionally reread it to refresh its ideas. Its existence in the world, as something he'd discuss and reference, would catalyze changes in his life.

———

In the morning, Tao bought another night at Union Hotel. He walked leisurely in sunlight smoking cannabis, eventually arriving at Valencia Whole Foods, a food store unrelated to Whole Foods, on Valencia and 21st, more stoned at around an hour after waking than he'd been in weeks or months. He crossed the street, sat on a raised area on the sidewalk, drank six eggs and a glass-bottled kombucha, researched directions to a public library, and returned his nearly depleted phone to Airplane Mode.

Walking north on Valencia, he began to fantasize about writing his book's epilogue. Kathleen had said many things he'd never heard before. He wanted to quote her at length. He was excited to selectively document spoken language, to share unusual fragments of dialogue, trialogue, syntax, and word choice by Kathleen, Finn, Klea, Paetra, Corinne, Chris, and others from the garden, in cars, on sidewalks, and in class. Because he'd unwittingly stopped the first two recordings, an unconscious selection of the possible material had already been made. This seemed auspicious. Tao had less audio than if he'd recorded straight through the first day, but, due to restarting twice, more Voice Memos, more variety.

Approaching 18th Street, he realized he couldn't find his phone. He checked his pockets unsystematically, feeling sometimes a little amused—checking some of his five pockets three or four times, it seemed—then checked each pocket in turn, finding no phone. The day before he'd lost his phone in his pocket, he knew.

He walked back to where he'd sat to drink eggs. The phone wasn't there. He sat where he'd sat and felt pleased by the warm sunlight, as he had before losing his phone. He walked where he'd walked, looking at the sidewalk for his phone. He entered three businesses, asked if anyone had turned in a phone, and they said no.

In Dolores Park, Tao lay on a slope of grass and felt, overall, glad his phone was gone. He looked forward to his phoneless day. In his notebook, he began writing the pros and cons of losing his phone and realized he'd lost all his photos and videos. With a pang of disappointment that made his heart beat faster—and with surprise he'd ignored or overlooked this until now—he realized he'd also lost all the Voice Memos:

- 1 hour 49 minutes with Kathleen in the library

- 6 minutes with Kathleen and Finn in the garden

- 2 minutes of Finn talking in the garden

- 40-something minutes of student introductions in the library

- 40-something minutes that included asking Finn two quantitative questions

He listed losing the photos, videos, and Voice Memos as the only cons. He felt worried. He reminded himself he'd posted two videos on Instagram and sent photos to his mom (he'd collect those later), then wrote these pros:

- Less mindless, repetitive, distracting, despair-causing, frustrating behavior

- Calmer thinking patterns/style

- Less things to focus on

- More focus on book

- Healthier for eyes

- Healthier for body

- Past abstinence has proven to have desirable effect on my life

- Closer to nature including more in-person interaction

- Different than before, a change, opportunity for evolution/variety

He added, obligatorily but, he felt, still helpfully, "Learning experience"—that he would, or could, learn from what had happened. He began wondering if he'd unconsciously gotten rid of his phone. After drinking eggs and kombucha, he'd carried their containers across the street with his right hand and put them in a metal trash can. Had his phone been in the same hand? Once, a year or two earlier, he'd tossed his phone into a makeshift trash bag in his room and retrieved it minutes later, surprised.

With excitement at a possible resolution—of having the Voice Memos again!—and a conflicted feeling of relinquishing the pros he'd collected into a substantial-seeming list, he returned to where he might have discarded his phone and saw the metal trash can had a comically thick, armor-like casing around it that was locked. He tried to search it, sticking his hand in a little, but the structure seemed designed to thwart him and he stopped.

Walking to the main branch of the public library, Tao noticed a row of camping tents—on the sidewalk across the street—in which people lived, apparently. Each tent on the wide-sidewalked block was paired with a tree, but not every tree had a tent. At an intersection, a man asked Tao for money and received. He thanked Tao and said someone had come out of a bar across the street and started "shit-talking" him for no reason. Stoned in public, Tao interacted with more people, often unconsciously reciprocating the calming, he felt, eye contact of panhandlers and homeless people.

Walking, he considered the cons of losing the Voice Memos. One con was that he'd inconvenienced Kathleen. Objective audio of what she'd said no longer existed. Tao wasn't sure what to do. Ask questions by email? Phone? Skype? Return to Occidental? He thought of when Kathleen noticed it was 3:00 P.M. and said time had gone fast—and that she had, at least twice, asked Tao if he was getting all the information he needed—and told himself she probably hadn't been too inconvenienced, but that, still, this was clumsy of him, to lose the precious Voice Memos—fatally clumsy, as a journalist and person. Journalists had done this to him before and then had repeated the same questions, which he didn't enjoy because, among other reasons, it underscored the situation's artificiality.

Arguing again against despair, Tao reminded himself he was very interested in Kathleen's thoughts, feelings, experiences, and knowledge and was writing about her, her family, and Botanical Dimensions in a book contracted to be published by Vintage, an imprint of Penguin Random House. Asking her to talk to him again about the same things in an interview format didn't seem too bad. This wasn't a newspaper or magazine assignment in which she'd be mechanically and disrespectfully reduced to an embarrassing and inaccurate headline, linking her non sequiturly to some absurd trend and then further labeling and categorizing her in promotional tweets and other language on various websites that future media, researching her, would repeat in slight variations indefinitely. This wasn't something Tao was belligerently and selfishly doing for a personal blog with a tiny readership in a misguided, "seize the day"–related disregard for Kathleen's time. It was for a book whose "positive and exploratory" tone Kathleen had said she appreciated, Tao reminded himself.

He considered the pros of losing the Voice Memos. Besides being a good learning experience, another pro was that this was an opportunity for his book to evolve. Another pro was that now he had an unusual and challenging task that interested and excited him and would require all his attention. His task was to remember the hundreds of minutes in Occidental when he believed his phone was recording—when, instead of trying to memorize everything, he'd tried to "be here now," as Kathleen quoted Ram Dass in her talks. He'd deliberately refrained from recalling those experiences—for, by now, one day and two nights—so they remained uniquely, he felt, undisturbed. Now he would go model them in prose.

In the library, using one of the two "express internet" computers, Tao went to iCloud.com/find and put his phone on Lost Mode, which, from what he could discern, wouldn't help since his phone had been on Airplane Mode. He reserved a seated computer to use from 3:00 P.M. to 4:00 P.M. He crossed the street and lay in sunny Civic Center Park, which was sparsely in use, mostly by alert, mobile, bored-seeming homeless people. From Tao's hundreds of book-related visits to cities across Earth since 2006, San Francisco at this time seemed to have the most homeless people.

Back in the library, seated with homeless people at one of the reservable computers with internet, Tao rapidly typed and edited and organized words and sentences about his time in Occidental. After his allotted hour, he went outside, smoked, stretched, and exercised, swinging his arms forward and back while walking. In his room and elsewhere, the past few years, he'd invented many exercises, naming and typing a little on each in notes.rtf. When he invented exercises, or personalized other aspects of life, he felt like an exclusive, non-recruiting cult.

Back in the library again, he sat in a chair in line for one of the unreservable "express internet" computers. He was second and last in line, then first and only. Then a man dressed like and as tall—at least six-five—and almost as muscular as an NBA basketball player sat by him and began talking to an imaginary person with whom, it seemed, he was in controlled, moderate, resolvable conflict. He had a lisp and smelled sour, like one of Tao's fermentations. Instead of sitting in one of the other three or four chairs, the man, who didn't seem to be waiting for a computer but just resting, had sat by Tao, but he seemed unaware of Tao—until after around five minutes, when he asked Tao to move his paper bag that was on the floor because it was "taking up too much space" and Tao moved it to his other side.

The man's complex natural sour smell helped Tao, who felt he'd benefit if he rubbed himself against or even licked the man's microbe-infested skin, which probably was relatively free of synthetic chemicals. In the past, Tao avoided sourness except in Sour Patch Kids, sweet and sour sauce, plastic packets of relish, and other substances he now viewed as toxic. Now he did not move to avoid natural sourness but enjoyed it physically and mentally. Compounds and microbes traveled invisibly from the lactic-acid fermenting man to Tao—who, as a twenty-first-century, computer-reliant human, was starved for plant, fungal, microbial, animal, and human contact—and then the library began closing and Tao and other people went outside.

The rest of the day and night, he walked through the city writing memories in his notebook while sometimes somewhat discreetly smoking cannabis, whose effects seemed as impressive and complicatedly magical as ever. He considered the possibility he was smoking cannabis that, for the first time in months, was not pesticide-ridden, as he suspected/assumed his illegal cannabis in New York was—cannabis he got by texting a number he'd forgotten how he'd gotten but seemed to have been using for years, then waiting one to eight hours until someone he only sometimes recognized arrived with cannabis. He downloaded recent memories into series of words, scrawling at one point that he felt "exquisitely, happily, discerningly stoned."

The next day was July 4. The library was closed. In a FedEx Office, at 35 cents per minute, Tao transferred notes from his notebook through his mind, where fragments became sentences, to the Google Drive document for his book's epilogue. Outside, he peed illegally behind a giant trash bin, then smoked cannabis, hurried inside, and continued working for around a half hour.

He walked to the harbor market and contemplated moderate exploration. He wanted to be moderately exploratory with, among other things, DMT. Applying patient, controlled, long-term effort in the DMT domain, he'd smoke it seven to fifteen more times in his life, and his accounts would appear in various forms in his oeuvre and the thirteen or however many DMT trips of Tao

Lin would be known and, he fantasized, could be analyzed and discussed like Chopin's twenty-one nocturnes or Lorrie Moore's thirty-eight short stories. His DMT trips, novels, short stories, and other sequences—in which each new entry was informed by a slightly larger history—would stabilize and complexify his life, leading him places he'd otherwise never go, he thought to himself while walking through the market.

Back in FedEx, he worked for another hour, finishing at 5:35 P.M. with 5,892 words. He printed the file, stapled the paper, and felt productive. He'd enjoyed it so much the previous night that he did it again: wandered the mostly unfamiliar city while becoming increasingly stoned, intermittently writing memories and ideas in his notebook. Walking circuitously to briefly explore, he encountered Rainbow Grocery, which he recognized from 2007, 2009, or 2010, he wasn't sure. He entered, browsed, bought nuts and seeds. He'd forgotten this place.

In Union Hotel, on the way to his room, Tao saw it was 8:07 P.M. on the digital clock behind the counter where the Indian family lived. Phoneless, he had a different relationship with time—which seemed good because he desired increased and varied familiarity with nanoseconds, microseconds, milliseconds, centiseconds, deciseconds, seconds, minutes, hours, days, weeks, months, years, decades, centuries, millennia, and other periods of time, like lunations, seasons, a million years, and a billion years.

In his room, he wrote about his day—that he'd transcribed his notes to a file and organized it into parts he could "enter and explore." He wrote that he was "smoking a small hit & going to sleep without alarm." Kneeling at the window, he blew cannabis smoke up and out and saw part of the twilight-blue sky.

He turned off the light and got into bed. There were fewer fireworks than he expected for the night of Independence Day. Manhattan was denser, he reminded himself, than San Francisco. He was in a large city, but he felt like he was in a suburban home, hearing sporadic fireworks elsewhere in the neighborhood. He focused on what he felt, and the feeling seemed surprisingly subtle. "I'm happier than I've ever been," he thought calmly. "Happier and healthier."

A few seconds later, he realized both how he would write his book's epilogue and how it would end, simultaneously and with clarity. He'd write it, he realized, as a short story—like the ones that had moved and consoled and inspired him in and after college—ending with him in bed thinking he was happier and healthier than he'd ever been! He'd quote his internal monologue, braiding life and literature for a long moment, a small paragraph.

He got out of bed, turned on the light, wrote a note to himself to write the epilogue as a short story ending with him thinking "happier and healthier," and returned to bed. Weeks later, working on the story, which had become novella-length, he'd notice that his sleepily stoned internal monologue had murmured language he'd in part absorbed, it seemed, from his mom, who in her email three days earlier had wished him "the best, healthiest and happiest birthday ever."

He fantasized about the myriad-seeming pros of this epilogue form—its holding capacity for a range of information, the option of third-person perspective, that he could insert ideas that didn't fit elsewhere, and the opportunity to end in a narrative, nonrhetorical, emotional moment—then stopped and focused on rest.

APPENDIX

1. There are ninety to one hundred natural types of atoms on Earth—hydrogen, helium, etc.

2. Most atoms aren't small, conceptually.

3. Oxygen is made of eight electrons, eight protons, eight neutrons.

4. Atoms automatically, in time, join to form molecules.

5. Hydrogen and oxygen form water, a 3-atom molecule.

6. Amino acids are a type of small molecule.

7. Amino acids are made by adding a "side chain" to a specific 9-atom molecule.

8. Glycine, a 10-atom amino acid, has a hydrogen atom as its side chain.

9. Tryptophan, a 27-atom amino acid, has an ethylene and an indole molecule.

10. Estimates of how many types of amino acids occur in biological systems range from hundreds to thousands, according to a 2013 paper in *Journal of Chemical Information and Modeling*.

11. But life uses only twenty different amino acids, made from ten to twenty-seven atoms, to build proteins. Francis Crick, co-discoverer of the structure of DNA, wrote in *Life Itself* (1981) that it was surprising only twenty were used and that it was the same twenty, made of only hydrogen, carbon, nitrogen, oxygen, and sulfur, for all life on Earth.

12. Life uses twenty-two amino acids, it has since been discovered, to build proteins, but the twenty-first and twenty-second—selenium-containing selenocysteine, used by animals but not fungi or land plants, and pyrrolysine, used by some bacteria—are inserted into proteins differently than the others.

13. Life is made of billions of types of proteins.

14. Life builds proteins by connecting tens to tens of thousands of amino acids in one-dimensional sequences that automatically fold, in microseconds, into three-dimensional objects that function by their unique shape. Before this was discovered in the twentieth century, no one seemed to have predicted it.

15. The dimensional inflation seems like the most surprising aspect of the process.

16. The others—atoms forming amino acids, forming proteins, forming cells—seem more predictable.

17. Proteins can't be made with atoms, only amino acids.

18. Titin, the largest known protein and third most abundant protein in adult human muscles, is made from 34,350 amino acids.

19. The smallest known foldable protein is the semi-synthetic, Gila monster saliva–derived Trp-Cage, which is twenty amino acids—NLYIQWLKDGGPSSGRPPPS—and looks like this when unfolded and folds in four microseconds:

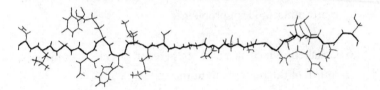

20. Hemoglobin, a protein that moves oxygen to tissues and carbon dioxide to lungs, is 574 amino acids.

21. Receptors are proteins. CB1 is 472 amino acids in humans. CB2 is 347, 360, and 361 amino acids in mice, humans, and rats.

22. CB1 and CB2 are two types of serpentine receptors, of which more than a thousand types exist in mammals and which cross the cell membrane seven times and are also called G-protein-coupled receptors.

23. Enzymes are proteins that accelerate chemical reactions. INMT is a 263–amino acid enzyme that can *N*-methylate tryptamine, which is decarboxylated tryptophan, twice to create *N,N*-dimethyltryptamine.

24. EPSPs is a 427–amino acid enzyme used by life in the seven-step shikimate pathway to create, among other compounds, phenylalaline, tyrosine, and tryptophan.

25. In March 2016, in their fifth paper on glyphosate, Samsel and Seneff theorized that life mistakenly inserts glyphosate instead of glycine into hundreds to thousands of proteins that depend on glycine to function, including EPSPs, the CYP enzymes, collagen, and various receptors, contributing to or causing autism, cancer, infertility, birth defects, diabetes, obesity, asthma, Alzheimer's, Crohn's, Parkinson's, and many other modern problems.

26. Collagen, which is 20 to 25 percent glycine, comprises a fourth of the proteins in humans.

27. There are "proteins whose job it is to unwind the double helix," wrote Crick.

28. A list of every known protein would begin with ones containing hundreds of atoms and end millions of entries later with titin, which contains more than 400,000 atoms.

29. On a different planet, the periodic table of elements would be the same, showing ninety-plus types of atoms, but a table of the planets' proteins would be much different.

30. This is because, I learned from Crick, on a different planet, life may have chosen a different set of twenty amino acids to use to build itself. Life that uses only sixteen amino acids probably exists on many of the hundreds of billions of plan-

ets in the Milky Way—and maybe these forms of life, lacking the complexity of twenty, never evolve past unicellular existence.

31. If we encountered a planet of life-forms made from twenty-eight amino acids, maybe they would seem, in a strange way, all the same—looking and acting in a certain 28–amino acid way. We would become self-conscious and realize that, despite our variety, from chlorella to flying fish to Barack Obama, we are almost all built from the same set of amino acids. Crick stressed that this was how terrestrial life was, beneath appearances, unified.

32. The knowledge of how to build proteins is stored in DNA. Human DNA codes for around twenty thousand proteins, each of which, post-assembly, can be modified up to a hundred ways.

33. Species know how to create unique sets of proteins, which partially determine their form.

34. DNA is made by connecting two small molecules, which are always the same, with a third, which can be adenine (fifteen atoms), guanine (sixteen atoms), thymine (fifteen atoms), or cytosine (thirteen atoms); each triplet is called a nucleotide.

35. DNA is read in three-nucleotide groups called codons. There are sixty-four codons because $4 \times 4 \times 4 = 64$.

36. Sixty-one codons refer to twenty amino acids; the other three mean "end chain" and can also refer to the twenty-first and

twenty-second amino acids. Tryptophan is the only amino acid of the main twenty with only one codon; the other nineteen have two to six codons.

37. Life reads a codon that says "adenine (A), adenine (A), guanine (G)" and knows to insert a lysine amino acid next, knowing as a planet knows how to orbit its star, by being its unique shape and following natural laws.

38. If I had a box of amino acid models and a model of twenty codons of DNA coding for Trp-Cage and I wanted to teach a child to build Trp-Cage, I would give the child a chart showing the twenty-two proteinogenic amino acids and "the genetic code."

39. The genetic code says what the codons mean—that GGA is glycine, UAA "end chain," etc.

40. Life does what the child would do—reads a codon, consults the code, inserts an amino acid, reads the next codon, etc.— automatically, using proteins and natural laws. It learned how over an unknown amount of time.

41. The automatic process involves transcription, translation, RNA, and ribosomes. "Because it is so complicated the reader should not attempt to struggle with all the details," wrote Crick.

42. The "important thing to realize," he felt, was that the genetic code "must have evolved from something much simpler."

43. Life built cells from proteins, animals from cells.

44. Life automatically, in time, created humans.

45. Crick pointed out that enough time—9.3 billion years—had already passed for life to have gone from "soup to man" twice by the time Earth formed. This made him theorize life began extraterrestrially and, over billions of years, spread to other stars and probably galaxies. Which made him theorize life on Earth was seeded from elsewhere, maybe as bacteria, which over three to four billion years became humans.

46. Humans created language.

47. English uses twenty-six letters, -,—, ;, :, ?, !, ., and other symbols, like ~, +, =, and ,.

48. Connecting words in a one-dimensional manner, with punctuation, humans created sentences. Instead of always folding the same way, like proteins, sentences dimensionally inflate in unique ways depending on the mind and time.

49. As life tunneled efflorescently through the universe into the imagination, complexity increased in a level-jumping, nonlinear manner.

50. Atoms, amino acids, proteins, cells, humans. Strokes, letters, words, sentences, books.

51. In 1937, Olaf Stapledon published *Star Maker*, a novel made of hundreds of thousands of symbols arranged one-dimensionally into thousands of sentences.

52. In *Star Maker*, a character in London goes outside one night

feeling discouraged and bleak, suddenly zooms away from Earth as a disembodied consciousness, and participates in the entire future history of the universe. At the end of the novel, the character, now comprised of every galaxy— around half—that had "awakened" sufficiently to form a mind, meets its creator.

53. The universe-character learns it's arguably Star Maker's first mature work. Requiring half a trillion years to sustain an incipient, cosmic mind for fifteen billion years, the universe was much more complex than Star Maker's earlier creations. Star Maker placed the half-conscious universe alongside its other art and, after contemplation, continued creating.

54. In April 1939, five months before the start of World War II, Jean Rhys published *Good Morning, Midnight*, a novel about a woman in her forties living in hotels in Paris in October 1937. It intimately conveyed the strange experience of being a lonely, afraid, alienated, modern, ideology-less human interacting with others in an unsatisfying manner.

55. It was in four parts, often used the ellipsis symbol, and included this sentence: "All that is left in the world is an enormous machine, made of white steel." And these: "I have another drink. Damned voice in my head, I'll stop you talking . . ."

56. In an interview with the *Paris Review* in 1979, Rhys said, "All of writing is a huge lake." She called herself one of the "mere trickles" and said, "All that matters is feeding the lake. I don't matter. The lake matters. You must keep feeding the lake."

57. Stapledon (1886–1950) and Rhys (1890–1979) are two of the 108 billion humans, according to the Population Reference Bureau, who've lived since 50,000 BC.

58. The effect of 108 billion humans metabolized on Earth over 52,000 years is agriculture, solitary confinement, skyscrapers, science fiction, postmodern novels, two world wars, factory farms, smoked DMT, ubiquitous glyphosate, computers, and the internet.

59. 108 billion molecules of LSD, the most potent psychedelic, metabolized in a human isn't noticeable.

60. 108 billion molecules of LSD weighs less than .0001 micrograms.

61. 150 micrograms of LSD are in an average, contemporary tab of LSD.

62. More than 225 million billion molecules are in 150 micrograms of LSD.

63. 225 million billion molecules of LSD metabolized in a human over hours is startlingly, scarily, and safely intense.

64. 225 million billion humans metabolized in a universe: ?

ACKNOWLEDGMENTS

Thank you to my family and friends; to Kathleen Harrison, Finn McKenna, and Klea McKenna; to Tim O'Connell, Bill Clegg, and Angie Venezia; and to my publisher, Vintage.

BIBLIOGRAPHY

INTRODUCTION

McKenna, Terence. "In Search of the Original Tree of Knowledge." Boulder, CO, May 29–31, 1992.

Narby, Jeremy. *The Cosmic Serpent: DNA and the Origins of Knowledge.* New York: Putnam, 1998.

WHY AM I INTERESTED IN HIM?

"A Conversation with Terence McKenna and Ram Dass (1992)." YouTube video, 40:05. October 1, 2011. https://www.youtube.com /watch?v=9Ih4Fg6P730.

McKenna, Terence. "Eros and the Eschaton." Kane Hall, University of Washington, Seattle, March 25, 1994.

———. "The World and Its Double." Nature Friends Lodge, Sierra Madre, CA, September 11, 1993.

Schopenhauer, Arthur. *The World as Will and Representation.* Translated by E. F. J. Payne. Mineola, NY: Dover Books, 1969.

TERENCE MCKENNA'S LIFE

Davis, Erik. "Terence McKenna's Last Trip." *Wired*, May 1, 2000.

"Ethnobotanist Discusses Her First DMT Experience." YouTube video, 2:10. January 10, 2010. https://www.youtube.com/watch?v= J8nYAogPw9w.

Kent, James. "Terence McKenna Interview, Part 1." *tripzine*, May 1, 2001. http://www.tripzine.com/listing.php?id=terence1.

McKenna, Dennis. *The Brotherhood of the Screaming Abyss: My Life with Terence McKenna*. St. Cloud, MN: Polaris Publications, 2012.

McKenna, Finn. Phone communication with author on Terence McKenna's biography, May 18, 2017.

McKenna, Klea. *The Butterfly Hunter*. Self-published, 2008.

McKenna, Terence. *Food of the Gods: The Search for the Original Tree of Knowledge—A Radical History of Plants, Drugs, and Human Evolution*. New York: Bantam Books, 1992.

———. "Logos Meets Eros." Wetland Preserves, New York, July 28, 1998.

———. "Packing for the Long Strange Trip." Starwood XIV, Sherman, NY, July 19, 1994.

———. "Psychedelics in the Age of Intelligent Machines" or "Shamans Among the Machines." Seattle, April 27, 1999.

———. *The Archaic Revival: Speculations on Psychedelic Mushrooms, the Amazon, Virtual Reality, UFOs, Evolution, Shamanism, the Rebirth of the Goddess, and the End of History*. San Francisco: HarperCollins, 1992.

———. *True Hallucinations: Being an Account of the Author's Extraordinary Adventures in the Devil's Paradise*. San Francisco: HarperCollins, 1993.

———. "Understanding and the Imagination in the Light of Nature." Los Angeles, October 17, 1987.

———, and Dennis McKenna. *The Invisible Landscape: Mind, Hallucinogens, and the I Ching*. New York: The Seabury Press, 1975.

Oss, O. T., and O. N. Oeric. *Psilocybin: Magic Mushroom Grower's Guide*. Berkeley: And/Or Press, 1976.

Miller, Sukie. "Terence McKenna." *Omni*, May 1993.

Schultes, Richard Evans. "Virola as an Orally Administered Hallucinogen." *Botanical Museum Leaflets* 22, no. 6 (June 25, 1969): 229–40.

Wasson, R. Gordon. "Seeking the Magic Mushroom." *Life*, June 10, 1957.

MY DRUG HISTORY

Doblin, Rick. "Pahnke's 'Good Friday Experiment': A Long-Term Follow-Up and Methodological Critique." *Journal of Transpersonal Psychology* 23, no. 1 (January 1991): 1–28.

Harrison, Kathleen. "The Perception of Feminine Personas in Psychedelic Species." Breaking Convention, London, July 12, 2015.

Lin, Tao. "Great American Novelist." *The Stranger*, September 23, 2010.

Moore, Lorrie. *Anagrams*. New York: Knopf, 1986.

———. *Birds of America*. New York: Knopf, 1998.

Ott, Jeff. *My World*. Van Nuys, CA: Subcity Records, 2000.

Pessoa, Fernando. *The Book of Disquiet*. Translated by Richard Zenith. New York: Penguin Classics, 2002.

Rhys, Jean. *Good Morning, Midnight*. London: Constable, 1939.

———. *Smile Please*. London: André Deutsch, 1979.

PSILOCYBIN

Azmitia, Efrain C. Email communication with the author on the age of serotonin, March 3, 2017.

———. "Evolution of Serotonin: Sunlight to Suicide." *Handbook of the Behavioral Neurobiology of Serotonin*. Edited by Christian Muller and Barry Jacobs. Cambridge, MA: Academic Press, 2009.

Bengtson, Stefan et al. "Fungus-like mycelial fossils in 2.4-billion-year-old vesicular basalt." *Nature Ecology & Evolution* 1, no. 0141 (April 24, 2017): 10.1038/s41559-017-0141.

Gallimore, Andrew. Facebook communication with the author on the age of DMT, April 4, 2017.

Haldane, J. B. S. *Possible Worlds and Other Papers*. London: Chatto & Windus, 1927.

Huxley, Aldous. *Heaven and Hell*. London: Chatto & Windus, 1956.

DMT

Burroughs, William S., and Allen Ginsberg. *The Yage Letters*. San Francisco: City Lights, 1963.

Gaffney, Elizabeth. "Lorrie Moore, The Art of Fiction No. 167." *Paris Review*, Spring/Summer 2001.

Gallimore, Andrew R., and David P. Luke. "DMT Research from 1956 to the Edge of Time." *Neurotransmissions: Essays on Psychedelics from Breaking Convention*. London: Strange Attractor Press, 2013.

Main, Douglas. "Glyphosate Now the Most-Used Agricultural Chemical Ever." *Newsweek*, February 2, 2016.

Price, Weston A. *Nutrition and Physical Degeneration*. New York: P. B. Hoeber, 1939.

Schultes, Richard Evans. *Where the Gods Reign: Plants and Peoples of the Colombian Amazon*. Sante Fe, NM: Synergetic Press, 1988.

Strassman, Rick. *DMT: The Spirit Molecule*. Rochester, VT: Park Street Press, 2000.

Szabo, Attila et al. "Psychedelic N,N-Dimethyltryptamine and 5-Methoxy-N,N-Dimethyltryptamine Modulate Innate and Adaptive Inflammatory Responses through the Sigma-1 Receptor of Human Monocyte-Derived Dendritic Cells." *PloS ONE* 9, no. 8 (August 2014): 10.1371/journal.pone.0106533.

———. "The Endogenous Hallucinogen and Trace Amine N,N-Dimethyltryptamine (DMT) Displays Potent Protective Effects against Hypoxia via Sigma-1 Receptor Activation in Human Primary iPSC-Derived Cortical Neurons and Microglia-Like Immune Cells." *Frontiers in Neuroscience* 10 (September 2016): 423.

SALVIA

Casselman, Ivan. "Genetics and Phytochemistry of *Salvia divinorum*." Ph.D thesis, Southern Cross University, May 26, 2016.

Harrison, Kathleen. "Folk Research: The Hidden Benefits of a Long Tradition." Psychedelic Science in the 21st Century, San Jose, CA, April 18, 2010.

———. "Indigenous Plant Wisdom." Entheobotany Conference, Palenque, Mexico, January 2001.

———. "Roads Where There Have Long Been Trails." *Terra Nova: Nature and Culture*, Summer 1998.

————. "Spirit in Nature: Psychedelic Plants and Mushrooms Through Native Eyes." World Psychedelic Forum, Basel, Switzerland, March 22, 2008.

————. "The Leaves of the Shepherdess." *Sisters of the Extreme: Women Writing on the Drug Experience.* Edited by Cynthia Palmer and Michael Horowitz. Park Street Press, 2000.

Jenks, Aaron et al. "Evolution and Origins of the Mazatec Hallucinogenic sage, *Salvia divinorum (Lamiaceae)*: A Molecular Phylogenetic Approach." *Journal of Plant Research* 124, no. 5 (September 2011): 593–600.

Ray, Thomas S. "Psychedelics and the Human Receptorome." *PloS ONE* 5, no. 3 (February 2010): 10.1371/journal.pone.0009019.

Sack, Kevin, and Brent McDonald. "Popularity of a Hallucinogen May Thwart Its Medical Uses." *New York Times*, September 8, 2008.

Seeman, Philip et al. "Dopamine D2(High) Receptors Stimulated by Phencyclidines, Lysergic Acid Diethylamide, Salvinorin A, and Modafinil." *Synapse* 63, no. 8 (August 2009): 698–704.

Siebert, Daniel J. "*Salvia divinorum* and Salvinorin A: New Pharmacologic Findings." *Journal of Ethnopharmacology* 43, no. 1 (June 1994): 53–56.

Soutar, Ian. "Ska Pastora—Leaves of the Shepherdess." *MAPS Bulletin* 11, no. 1 (Spring 2001): 32–37.

Viebrock, Susan. "Ethnobotanist Kathleen Harrison at Shroomfest 2012." *Telluride Inside*, August 15, 2012.

WHY ARE PSYCHEDELICS ILLEGAL?

Baum, Dan. "Legalize It All: How to Win the War on Drugs." *Harper's*, April 2016.

Collins, Anne. *In the Sleep Room: The Story of the CIA Brainwashing Experiments in Canada.* Toronto: Lester and Orpen Dennys Ltd., 1988.

Duvall, Chris. *Cannabis.* London: Reaktion Books, 2015.

Eisler, Riane. *The Chalice and the Blade: Our History, Our Future.* New York: Harper & Row, 1987.

Frood, Arran. "Cluster Busters." *Nature Medicine*, December 28, 2006.

Gimbutas, Marija. *The Language of the Goddess: Unearthing the Hidden Symbols of Western Civilization.* New York: Thames and Hudson, 1989.

————, with Miriam Robbins Dexter. *The Living Goddesses.* Berkeley: University of California Press, 1999.

Halpern, John H., and Harrison G. Pope Jr. "Do Hallucinogens Cause Residual Neuropsychological Toxicity?" *Drug and Alcohol Dependence* 53, no. 3 (February 1999): 247–56.

Hersh, Seymour M. "Huge C.I.A. Operation Reported in U.S. Against Antiwar Forces, Other Dissidents in Nixon Years." *New York Times,* December 22, 1974.

Hofmann, Albert. *LSD: My Problem Child.* New York: McGraw-Hill, 1980.

Horowitz, Michael. "Interview: Albert Hofmann." *High Times* 11, July 1976.

Ignatieff, Michael. "C.I.A.; What Did the C.I.A. Do to His Father?" *New York Times Magazine,* April 1, 2001.

Lee, Martin A. *Smoke Signals: A Social History of Marijuana—Medical, Recreational and Scientific.* New York: Simon & Schuster, 2012.

May, Peter. "Cluster Headache, Dreaming & Neurogenesis." Self-published, 2006. http://www.scribd.com/document/128681079/CH-Dreaming-Neurogenesis.

McKenna, Terence. "Nature Is the Center of the Mandala." Shared Visions, Berkeley, September 12, 1987.

Mellaart, James. *Çatal Hüyük: A Neolithic Town in Anatolia.* New York: McGraw-Hill, 1967.

————. *Earliest Civilizations of the Near East.* New York: McGraw-Hill, 1965.

Pollan, Michael. "The Trip Treatment." *New Yorker,* February 9, 2015.

Rabin, Roni Caryn. "More Overdose Deaths from Anxiety Drugs." *New York Times,* February 25, 2016.

Ruck, Carl A. P. *Sacred Mushrooms of the Goddess: Secrets of Eleusis.* Berkeley: Ronin Publishing, 2006.

Stone, Merlin. *When God Was a Woman.* New York: Dial Press, 1976.

U.S. Congress. *Joint Hearing Before the Select Committee on Intelligence and the Subcommittee on Health and Scientific Research of the Com-*

mittee on Human Resources on Project MKULTRA, the CIA's Program of Research in Behavioral Modification. Hearings. 95th Cong., 1st sess., August 3, 1977.

Wasson, R. Gordon, Albert Hofmann, and Carl Ruck. *The Road to Eleusis: Unveiling the Secret of the Mysteries.* San Diego: Harcourt, Brace, Jovanovich, 1978.

CANNABIS

Almécija, Sergio et al. "The Femur of *Orrorin tugenensis* Exhibits Morphometric Affinities with Both Miocene Apes and Later Hominins." *Nature Communications* 4 (December 2013): 2888.

Ambrose, Stanley H. "Late Pleistocene Human Population Bottlenecks, Volcanic Winter, and Differentiation of Modern Humans." *Journal of Human Evolution* 34, no. 6 (June 1998): 623–51.

Christenhusz, Maarten J. M., and James W. Byng. "The Number of Known Plants Species in the World and Its Annual Increase." *Phytotaxa* 261, no. 3 (April 2016): 201–17.

Crane, Peter. *Ginkgo: The Tree That Time Forgot.* New Haven, CT: Yale University Press, 2013.

Gertsch, Jürg et al. "Phytocannabinoids Beyond the *Cannabis* Plant—Do They Exist?" *British Journal of Pharmacology* 160, no. 3 (June 2010): 523–29.

Harrison, Kathleen. "Psychedelic Insight: Bringing It Back to Social Reality." Entheo-Health and Wellness Forum, CIIS, San Francisco, December 13, 2013.

———. "Who Is Cannabis? Her Persona & Role in Personal & Cultural Experience." Visionary Conference, Los Angeles, September 26, 2015.

Hazard, John. "Terence McKenna's Final Earthbound Interview." *Reality Sandwich*, October 1998.

Hublin, Jean-Jacques et al. "New Fossils from Jebel Irhoud, Morocco and the Pan-African Origin of *Homo sapiens.*" *Nature* 546, no. 7657 (June 2017): 289–92.

Iversen, Leslie. *The Science of Marijuana.* New York: Oxford University Press, 2008.

Jacobson, Mark. "Is Terence McKenna the Brave Prophet of the Next Psychedelic Revolution, or Is His Cosmic Egg Just a Little Bit Cracked?" *Esquire*, June 1992.

Keltner, Dacher, and Jonathan Haidt. "Approaching Awe, a Moral, Spiritual, and Aesthetic Emotion." *Cognition and Emotion* 17, no. 2 (March 2003): 297–314.

Malaspinas, Anna-Sapfo et al. "A Genomic History of Aboriginal Australia." *Nature* 538, no. 7624 (October 2016): 207–14.

Mandelbrot, Benoit. *The Fractal Geometry of Nature*. New York: W. H. Freeman and Company, 1982.

McKenna, Terence. "I Understand Philip K. Dick." *In Pursuit of Valis: Selections from the Exegesis*. Edited by Lawrence Sutin. Nevada City: Underwood Books, 1991.

———, Ralph Abraham, and Rupert Sheldrake. "Cannabis Trialogue." Esalen Institute, Big Sur, CA, 1991.

Morris, Hamilton, Daniel Pinchbeck, and Adam Green. "Art, Drugs & Consciousness." The Intercourse, Brooklyn, NY, October 25, 2012.

Schopenhauer, Arthur. *Parerga and Paralipomena*. Translated by E. F. J. Payne. New York: Oxford University Press, 1974.

Schwartz, Oscar. "Giving Tao Lin Good Quality Marijuana in Melbourne, Australia After Reading a Tweet Tao Lin Wrote in Brisbane, Australia About His Desire for Marijuana." *Scum*, December 21, 2013.

Shiota, Michelle N. et al. "Positive Emotion Dispositions Differentially Associated with Big Five." *Journal of Positive Psychology* 1, no. 2 (April 2006): 61–71.

Stellar, Jennifer et al. "Positive Affect and Markers of Inflammation: Discrete Positive Emotions Predict Lower Levels of Inflammatory Cytokines." *Emotion* 15, no. 2 (April 2015): 129–33.

Storey, Michael et al. "Astronomically Calibrated 40Ar/39Ar Age for the Toba Supereruption and Global Synchronization of Late Quaternary Records." *Proceedings of the National Academy of Sciences of the United States of America* 109, no. 46 (November 2012): 18684–88.

Zeder, Melinda. "The Origins of Agriculture in the Near East." *Current Anthropology* 52, no. S4 (October 2011): S221–35.

EPILOGUE

Adams, Kelly M. et al. "Status of Nutrition Education in Medical Schools." *American Journal of Clinical Nutrition* 84, no. 4 (April 2006): 941S–944S.

Anderson, M. Kat. *Tending the Wild: Native American Knowledge and the Management of California's Natural Resources.* Berkeley: University of California Press, 2006.

Benbrook, Charles M. "Trends in Glyphosate Herbicide Use in the United States and Globally." *Environmental Sciences Europe* 28, no. 3 (February 2016): 10.1186/s12302-016-0070-0.

Bowman, Katy. *Move Your DNA: Restore Your Health Through Natural Movement.* Sequim, WA: Propriometrics Press, 2014.

Browne, Hilary P. et al. "Culturing of 'Unculturable' Human Microbiota Reveals Novel Taxa and Extensive Sporulation." *Nature* 533, no. 7604 (May 2016): 10.1038/nature17645.

Carson, Rachel. *Silent Spring.* New York: Houghton Mifflin, 1962.

Chen, Ellen Marie. "Tao as the Great Mother and the Influence of Motherly Love in the Shaping of Chinese Philosophy." *History of Religions* 14, no. 1 (August 1974): 51–64.

Davis, Erik. "Botanical Beings: A Talk with Ethnobotanist Kathleen Harrison." *Expanding Mind*, May 14, 2015.

De Angelis, Maria et al. "*Lactobacillus rossiae*, a Vitamin B12 Producer, Represents a Metabolically Versatile Species within the Genus *Lactobacillus*." *PLoS ONE* 9, no. 9 (September 2014): 10.1371/journal .pone.0107232.

Fallon, Sally, with Mary G. Enig. *Nourishing Traditions: The Cookbook that Challenges Politically Correct Nutrition and Diet Dictocrats.* Washington, DC: NewTrends Publishing, 1995.

"Glyphosate Found in Major Childhood Vaccines: Moms & Scientists Demand CDC & FDA Test Vaccines for Glyphosate." Moms Across America, Press Release, September 6, 2016.

Hammerschlag, Carl Allen. "The Huichol Offering: A Shamanic Healing Journey." *Journal of Religion & Health* 48, no. 2 (June 2009): 246–58.

Harrison, Kathleen. "Treat Her Right: Lessons from a Medicine Walk." *MAPS Bulletin* 19, no. 1 (Spring 2009): 8–11.

Honeycutt, Zen. "Glyphosate in Vaccines Report." Moms Across America, Press Release, September 5, 2016.

Janušonis, Skirmantas. "Functional Associations among G Protein-Coupled Neurotransmitter Receptors in the Human Brain." *BMC Neuroscience* 15, no. 16 (January 2014): 10.1186/1471-2202-15-16.

Jones, Marie D., and John Savino. *Supervolcano: The Catastrophic Event That Changed the Course of Human History*. Wayne, NJ: New Page Books, 2007.

"Kathleen Harrison: LSD Didn't Really Prepare Me for DMT." YouTube video, 1:14. September 26, 2011. https://www.youtube.com/watch?v=DuU_qMTuJWw.

Katz, Sandor. *Wild Fermentation: The Flavor, Nutrition, and Craft of Live-Culture Foods*. White River Junction, VT: Chelsea Green Publishing, 2003.

Kresser, Chris. "HLA-B27 and Autoimmune Disease: Is a Low-Starch Diet the Solution?" ChrisKresser.com, July 21, 2016.

Lin, J. T. In-person communication with the author on the lens of the human eye, March 15, 2017.

Lin, Yuchin. Email communication with the author on tone in Mandarin, June 29, 2017.

Lloyd-Price, Jason et al. "The Healthy Human Microbiome." *Genome Medicine* (2016): 10.1186/s13073-016-0307-y.

Majewski, Michael S. et al. "Pesticides in Mississippi Air and Rain: A Comparison between 1995 and 2007." *Environmental Toxicology and Chemistry* 33, no. 6 (June 2014): 1283–93.

McDougle, Daniel R. et al. "Anti-Inflammatory ω-3 Endocannabinoid Epoxides." *Proceedings of the National Academy of Sciences of the United States of America* 114, no. 30 (July 2017): E6034–43.

Mercurio, Philip et al. "Glyphosate Persistence in Seawater." *Marine Pollution Bulletin* 85, no. 2 (August 2014): 385–90.

Oudin, Anne et al. "Association between Neighbourhood Air Pollution Concentrations and Dispensed Medication for Psychiatric Disorders in a Large Longitudinal Cohort of Swedish Children and Adolescents." *BMJ Open* 6, no. 6 (June 2016): e010004.

Samsel, Anthony, and Stephanie Seneff. "Glyphosate's Suppression of Cytochrome P450 Enzymes and Amino Acid Biosynthesis by the Gut Microbiome: Pathways to Modern Diseases." *Entropy* 15, no. 4 (April 2013): 1416–63.

Schnorr, Stephanie L. et al. "Gut Microbiome of the Hadza Hunter-Gatherers." *Nature Communications* (April 2014): 10.1038/ncomms 4654.

Scribner, Elisabeth A. et al. "Concentrations of Glyphosate, Its Degradation Product, Aminomethylphosphonic Acid, and Glufosinate in Ground- and Surface-Water, Rainfall, and Soil Samples Collected in the United States, 2001–06." U.S. Geological Survey, Scientific Investigations Report 2007-5122.

Sender, Ron, Shai Fuchs, and Ron Milo. "Revised Estimates for the Number of Human and Bacteria Cells in the Body." *PloS Biology* 14, no. 8 (August 19, 2016): 10.1371/journal.pbio.1002533.

Singer, Katie. *An Electronic Silent Spring: Facing the Dangers and Creating Safe Limits.* Great Barrington, MA: Portal Books, 2014.

Sonnenburg, Erica D. et al. "Diet-induced Extinctions in the Gut Microbiota Compound Over Generations." *Nature* 529, no. 7585 (January 2016): 212–15.

United States Department of Agriculture. "Pesticide Data Program: Annual Summary, Calendar Year 2015." November 2016.

U.S. Geological Survey. "Common Weed Killer Is Widespread in the Environment." Environmental Health—Toxic Substances Hydrology Program, April 23, 2014.

Zelano, Christina et al. "Nasal Respiration Entrains Human Limbic Oscillations and Modulates Cognitive Function." *Journal of Neuroscience* 36, no. 49 (December 2016): 12448–67.

APPENDIX

Crick, Francis. *Life Itself.* New York: Simon & Schuster, 1981.

Linke, Wolfgang A., and N. Hamdani. "Gigantic Business: Titin Functions in Health and Disease." *Circulation Research* 114, no. 6 (March 2014): 1052–68.

Meringer, Markus et al. "Beyond Terrestrial Biology: Charting the Chemical Universe of α-Amino Acid Structures." *Journal of Chemical Information and Modeling* 53, no. 11 (October 2013): 2851–62.

Ponomarenko, Elena A. et al. "The Size of the Human Proteome: The Width and Depth." *International Journal of Analytical Chemistry* 2016 (April 2016): 10.1155/2016/7436849.

Psilo, Earth, Spoon. "Ask Erowid: ID 3083: How Many LSD Molecules in a Hit of LSD?" Erowid.org, December 27, 2004.

Qiu, Linlin et al. "Smaller and Faster: The 20-Residue Trp-Cage Protein Folds in 4 μs." *Journal of the American Chemical Society* 124, no. 44 (October 2002): 12952–53.

Samsel, Anthony, and Stephanie Seneff. "Glyphosate Pathways to Modern Diseases V: Amino Acid Analogue of Glycine in Diverse Proteins." *Journal of Biological Physics and Chemistry* 16 (March 2016): 9–46.

Seneff, Stephanie. "Glyphosate and Collagen: Widespread Consequences." *Wise Traditions in Food, Farming and the Healing Arts* 17, no. 4 (Winter 2016): 34–40.

Stapledon, Olaf. *Star Maker*. London: Methuen Publishing Ltd., 1937.

Vreeland, Elizabeth. "Jean Rhys, The Art of Fiction No. 64." *Paris Review*, Fall 1979.

LEAVE SOCIETY
BY TAO LIN

A bold portrait of a writer working to balance all his lives—as an artist, a son, and a loner.

In 2014, a novelist named Li leaves Manhattan to visit his parents in Taipei for ten weeks. He doesn't know it yet, but his life will begin to deepen and complexify on this trip. As he flies between these two worlds—year by year, over four years—he will flit in and out of optimism, despair, loneliness, sanity, bouts of chronic pain, and drafts of a new book. He will incite and temper arguments, uncover secrets about nature and history, and try to understand how to live a meaningful life as an artist and a son. But how to fit these pieces of his life together? Where to begin? Or should he leave society altogether?

In his most recent work, Tao Lin delivers an engrossing and hopeful novel about life, fiction, and where the two blur together that builds toward a stunning, if unexpected, romance. Exploring everyday events and scenes—waiting rooms, dog walks, family meals—while investigatively venturing to the edges of society, where culture dissolves into mystery, Lin spins the ordinary into something monumental and shows what it is to write a novel in real time. Illuminating and deeply felt, *Leave Society* is a masterly story about life and art at the end of history.